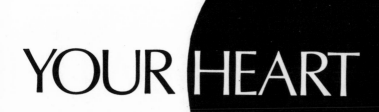

YOUR HEART

Copyright © Ottawa 1975 by Optimum Publishing Company Limited and Arthur Vineberg & Company Reg'd.

Published by Optimum Publishing Company Limited, 245 rue St-Jacques, Montreal, Quebec, Canada H2Y 1M6.

Published simultaneously in the United States by Quadrangle/ The New York Times Book Company, 10 East 53 Street, New York, New York 10022.

Illustrated by Garry Hamilton

Printed and bound in Canada

Library of Congress Cataloging in Publication Data

Vineberg, Arthur Martin, 1903-
    How to live with your heart.

    Bibliography: p.
    1. Heart—Diseases.   2. Heart—Diseases
—Prevention.   3. Heart—Surgery.   I. Title.
RC672.V56   616.1'2'05   74-25204
ISBN 0-8129-0549-0

How To Live With Your Heart

QUADRANGLE

The New York Times Book Co.

The Family
Guide To
Heart Health

by Arthur Vineberg, M.D.

HOW TO LIVE WITH

CONTENTS

Chapter   **Page**

1   You Owe It to Your Family to Read This Book   11

2   Your Heart—How It Works   36

3   Diagnosis—The Heart Attack   44

4   Stress—The Rat Race and Your Heart   61

5   Sex and Your Heart   78

6   Food and Your Heart   86

7   Exercise and Your Heart   96

8   Heart Surgery I—The Vineberg Procedure   108

9   Heart Surgery II—Revascularization and Other Procedures 134

10   Your Heart and the Family Tree   151

Appendix A—Resuscitation   157

Appendix B—Cholesterol and Calorie Diet Chart   162

Appendix C—Exercise Chart   190

The Heart Dictionary   195

Bibliography and Sources   215

ACKNOWLEDGMENTS

How To Live With Your Heart offers a family program for the care of the heart. In the surgical chapters it describes operations which I developed in the department of experimental surgery at McGill University, starting in 1946, and some others developed in other North American centers. All the operations at McGill were laboratory-tested for two to five years before the procedures were adopted in the treatment of human coronary artery obstructive disease, the first patient being operated on at the Royal Victoria Hospital in Montreal in 1950.

What we have achieved has been made possible by the co-operation of a great many people, not only at McGill University and the Royal Victoria Hospital but at medical centers throughout Canada and the United States.

Particularly helpful to me have been Dr. Hebel Hoff, former Professor of Physiology, McGill University, now in Texas, who examined my first successful implant and attested to its success; Dr. Henry MacIntosh, who determined how much blood the internal mammary artery was capable of delivering to an animal's heart; and the late Dr. Lyman Duff, Professor of Pathology at McGill and the R.V.H., who documented the experimental work and encouraged me, after five years, to apply to human beings what was then an experimental operation for the treatment of coronary artery insufficency.

I am indebted to Dr. G. C. McMillan, Professor of Pathology at McGill University and the R.V.H., and his successor, Dr. W. J. Pirozynski, and to Dr. Sergio A. Bencosme, who proved that the internal mammary artery actually set up real arterial branches. I also

6

acknowledge the support given by Dr. Walter Scriver, Professor of Medicine at McGill and Director of the Department of Medicine at R.V.H. He appointed Drs. Phillip Hill and Peter Pare, of the department, to select and care for my patients, thus initiating a surgical-medical team in the early 1950s.

These excellent physicians were succeeded by Dr. John Shanks, cardiologist at the R.V.H., with whom I have been associated for many years in the selection and care of coronary patients requiring surgery. Throughout the years, he has been a keen supporter of my revascularization surgery, as has Dr. Maurice McGregor, Professor of Medicine at McGill and Director of Medicine at the R.V.H.

In the Department of Surgery, I acknowledge the active support of the late Dr. Gavin Miller, Professor of Surgery at McGill and Chief of Surgery at the R.V.H., and his successor, Dr. Donald Webster, and Dr. Lloyd D. MacLean, present Director of Surgery at R.V.H., as well as that of Dr. Anthony Dobell now Surgeon-in-Chief at the Montreal Children's Hospital, Professor of the Department of Surgery, R.V.H., and Director of the division of cardiovascular and thoracic surgery at McGill.

I wish to acknowledge in addition the support that was and still is given to me by my French-Canadian confreres; in particular Doctors Edward Gagnon and Paul David who invited me to work at the Institut De Cardiologie De Montreal in the late 1950's and for their continued support of arterial implant revascularization surgery.

I am greatly indebted to the Royal Victoria's Department of Anesthesia under Dr. Philip Bromage, whose associates, Dr. Arthur Sheridan and Dr. John E. Wynands, have never turned down a patient because he was too ill. Utilizing their great skills, these dedicated men have managed to anesthetize patients with some of the most advanced cases of coronary artery disease, many of them rejected by other medical centers because they were considered too ill to undergo surgery.

More than thirty young men have trained with me and have aided in the development of various revascularization operations. Twenty-two of them received their Master of Science degrees under my direction at McGill, and many of my one-time students, now doctors or surgeons in other parts of the world, are staunch advocates of my method of revascularization surgery.

Much support has come from my surgical and medical confreres in Canada and the United States. The three to whom I am foremost indebted are the late Dr. Paul Dudley White, Chief of the

Cardiac Unit, the Massachusetts General Hospital and Dr. Mason Sones, director of the Cardiac Catheterization Department of the Cleveland Clinic, Cleveland, Ohio. Dr. Sones performed an angiogram on one of my 7½-year-old internal mammary artery implants in 1961 which showed it to be open and working. The third from whom I have received continuous support is Dr. Donald Effler, Director of the Department of Cardiovascular and Thoracic Surgery, Cleveland Clinic, who has actively performed mammary artery implants and continuously has supported the principle of implant surgery. Dr. Wilfred G. Bigelow, Director of the Department of Cardiovascular and Thoracic Surgery, Toronto General Hospital, Toronto, Ontario has been and still is actively implanting internal mammary arteries; and Dr. Wilbert Keon, Head of the Department of Cardiovascular and Thoracic Surgery, Ottawa Civic Hospital, Ottawa, Ontario, is a most ardent supporter of my method of surgery, which he uses jointly with aorto-coronary vein bypass grafts. Dr. G. David Hooper, thoracic surgeon, has performed a large series of implants which have been studied and evaluated by Dr. G. Fitzgibbon, cardiologist, of the National Defence Medical Center, Ottawa, Ontario. Dr. William Bloomer, thoracic surgeon of St. Mary's Hospital, Long Beach, California also has a long-term series of implants which he is still performing successfully.

I am indebted, too, to Dr. Alton Ochsner, founder and Surgeon-in-Chief of the Ochsner Clinic, New Orleans; Dr. Paul David, Executive Director of the Institute of Cardiology of Montreal; Dr. Goffrado Gensini, Director of St. Joseph's Hospital Health Center, and The MSgr. Toomey, Cardiovascular Laboratory and Research Department, Syracuse, New York, and to his surgical associate, Dr. Ernest J. Delmonico, Jr., thoracic surgeon.

I shall also be eternally grateful for the twenty-four-hour support of the Royal Victoria Hospital Department of Nursing, which has been one of our most important aids in handling far-advanced cases of coronary artery disease. I would also like to acknowledge the support of Douglas J. MacDonald, Executive Director, Royal Victoria Hospital.

Our research has been most generously supported through the years at first by the Department of Public Health and Welfare of Canada and then by the Medical Research Council of Canada, and by Mr. Nathan Cummings and Mr. Stanley Vineberg, my brother.

Finally, I would like to express my gratitude to Bill Trent and Michael S. Baxendale who collaborated with me in the writing and preparation of this book.

For my wife Ann.

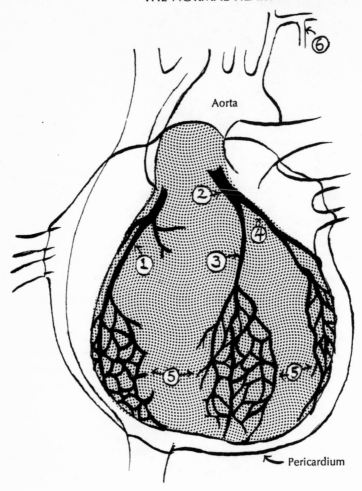

Aorta

Pericardium

Fig. 1. (1) Right coronary artery
(2) Left coronary artery
(3) Anterior descending artery
(4) Circumflex artery
(5) Myocardial arterioles
(6) Left internal mammary artery

CHAPTER 1

You Owe It to Your Family to Read This Book

John Blackburn is a big, rugged, heavy-set man with broad shoulders, strong hands, and the wrinkled, leathery kind of face that tells you he's worked outdoors all of his life. Looking at him, you'd find it hard to believe that he once had a heart condition so severe he couldn't even walk to the corner.

John is one of my pioneer patients of the early 1950s. He was part of the first concrete evidence that surgery could be the answer to an ailing heart. He became the proof positive that a heart attack needn't cripple a man for life. He was in a very real sense one of the shining hopes in the then fledgling world of heart surgery.

In the story of John there is a message for the 25 million North Americans currently afflicted with diseases of the heart and coronary arteries. The message: there is *hope*.

John is by no means unique. There are thousands of people, who were near death at one time or another, now playing golf, swimming, riding horses, digging wells, driving trucks, and generally living normal lives after surgery. But John was one of the first —and perhaps that fact alone qualifies him for special mention.

I can still see him in a ward in Montreal's Royal Victoria Hospital. He was a big, affable Californian, his physical strength drained, his once sun-bronzed face now ashen, snatching quick,

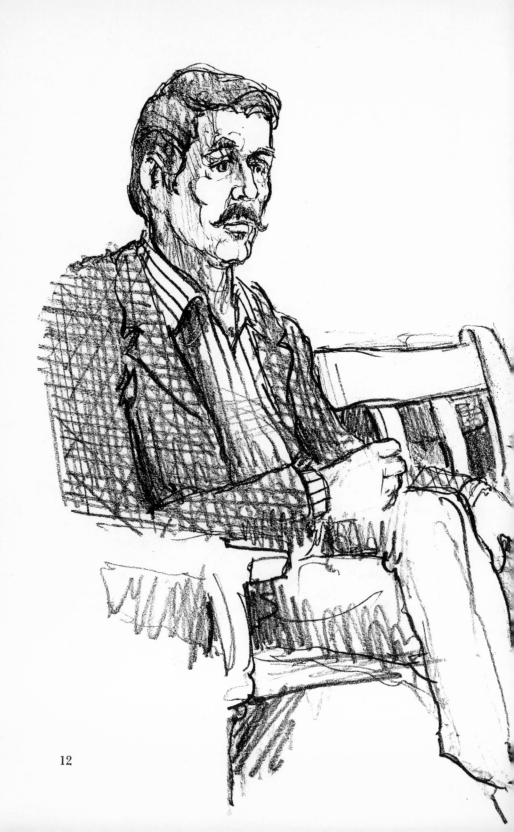

12

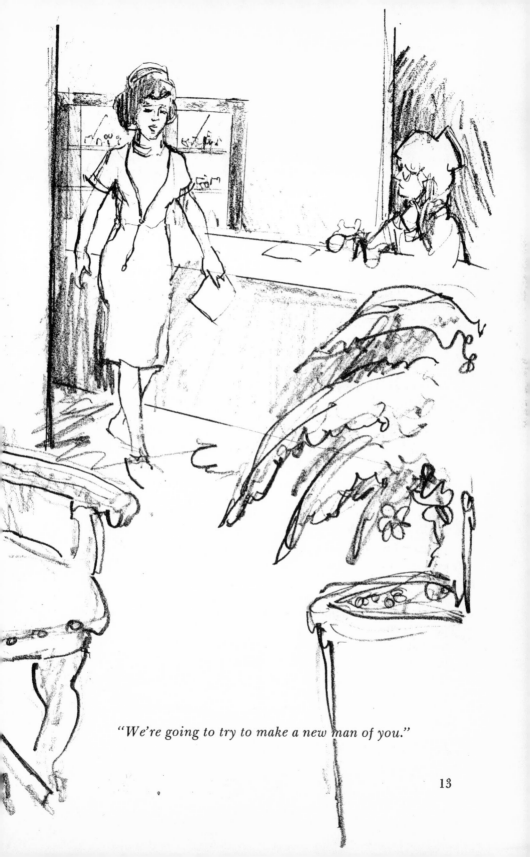

"We're going to try to make a new man of you."

uneven gulps of air, pursing his lips in anticipation of pain.

He wanted the answer to the two questions every person facing surgery asks: first, what were his chances and second, what precisely was I going to do to him.

That was in December 1953. In those days there were a good many skeptics, and they didn't mind saying that a surgeon had to be a little crazy to think he could implant an artery into a human heart and direct a fresh new supply of blood into it.

What were his chances? I pondered the matter for some time. I had an operation in mind for him. It was one I had developed—the mammary artery implant—but only two surgeons in the whole world were performing it. I was one. The other was Dr. Wilfred G. Bigelow, of Toronto, who had learned the procedure from me. We were just starting out and didn't know then what we know today. So, telling a patient that he could expect this, that, or the other thing was something we couldn't do.

Instead, I answered his second question. "We're going to try to make a new man of you," I said.

This was an entirely truthful remark. That was exactly what we intended to do: we were going to *try* to make a new man of him. We had had hundreds of successful tests with animals and even some successful human implants, so we knew pretty well what we could accomplish. But still, we had barely crossed the threshold.

John came to me in a roundabout way. In the summer of 1953, I had spoken in Los Angeles on the implant operation, and John's wife, Catherine, had read about it in the newspapers. She was desperate. In July 1952, John had had a heart attack. It had come suddenly, a violent, crushing pain in the chest. He spent seven weeks in hospital, then went home. After a day at home he returned to hospital for another five weeks. The results were unsatisfactory. Now, a year later, he was in almost constant pain. He couldn't walk more than a block.

Catherine wrote me, spelling out the danger signals like the careful observer she had become. If John were up long, he got a pain in the chest and down the back of his left arm. He had pain even at rest and shortness of breath after exertion. Catherine wanted to bring him to me, nearly four thousand miles away in Montreal. The local doctors were unable to help him. In fact, they didn't seem to know *what* to do.

At the Royal Victoria Hospital, John told a cardiologist about himself. He was 40, though he looked 50. He had once been a light heavyweight fighter in the United States Army. He had had vague

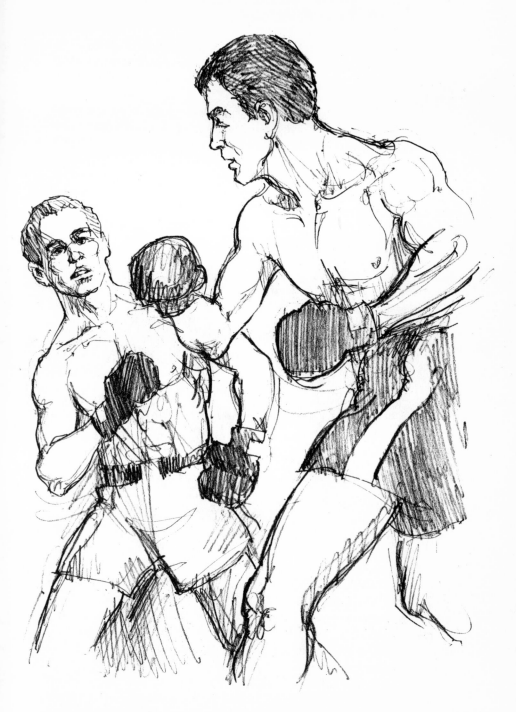

He had once been a light heavyweight fighter in the U.S. Army.

LEFT VENTRICULAR INTERNAL
MAMMARY ARTERY IMPLANT
(Vineberg Operation)

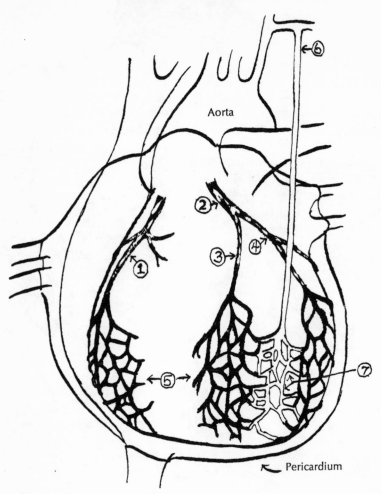

Fig. 2. (1) Diseased right coronary artery
(2) Diseased left coronary artery
(3) Diseased anterior descending coronary artery
(4) Diseased circumflex coronary artery
(5) Non-diseased myocardial arterioles
(6) Non-diseased left internal mammary artery
(7) New branches of internal mammary artery
implanted in heart muscle.

minor chest pains most of his life but every physician who had seen him had ascribed the pain to pleurisy.

We didn't talk about coronary profiles in those days but we knew that John had had two strikes against him before his attack. First, he had been overweight, tipping the scales at 230 pounds. This was heavy even for a six-footer. Second, he had a family history of heart disease, and we recognized that heredity played a role in the disease. His mother and a brother had both died of it.

The cardiologist made his diagnosis. John had progressive coronary heart disease. One, two, perhaps all three arteries—the pipelines through which blood travels to the heart—may have become blocked, or so narrowed by cholesterol and calcium deposits that the blood had difficulty reaching its destination. John was one of many millions of North Americans who had begun to develop coronary artery disease early—as early as their teenage years.

An electrocardiogram showed evidence of an old scar in the front of the heart, presumably the result of John's attack of the previous year. A later examination disclosed a narrowing of the arteries behind the eyes due to atherosclerosis.

We decided he should undergo revascularization surgery which, stated in simple terms, meant that the blood supply to his heart would be re-established by means of an artery grafted directly into the heart muscle. A sophisticated medical plumbing job—to run a new pipeline into the patient's heart. (Fig. 2).

Since 1945, working at the Department of Experimental Surgery at McGill University in Montreal, I had tested many methods of introducing new sources of oxygenated blood into the heart. By now, however, it was clear to me that the answer lay with the patient's own internal mammary arteries, located below the breast bone. (They are known as mammaries because, in the female, they supply blood to the breasts or mamma, and to the chest muscles which lie beneath the breasts, known as pectoral muscles. In the male they are larger than in the female because of the larger size of the male chest or pectoral muscles.)

The heart, considered a sacrosanct organ by some religious thinkers through the centuries—some thought it was the seat of the soul—was still relatively unexplored surgical territory. It was not until 1950 that anyone had put new arteries into the wall of the hard-working left ventricular human pump, as I had done in that year. There was great fear that the heart would stop during the surgery. Some surgeons had worked inside heart chambers, attempting to correct holes in the heart in babies and young children. No

THE OPERATION—STEP 1

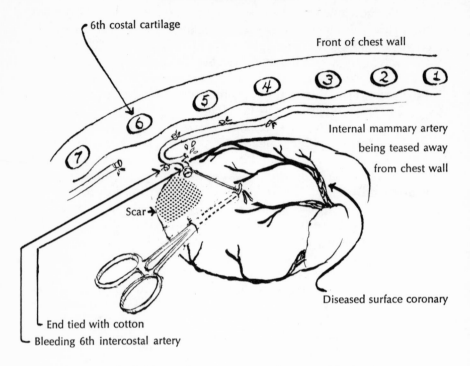

Fig. 3. The left internal mammary artery is prepared for implantation into the left ventricular wall.

one, however, had dared do what I was about to do—make a tunnel in the wall of the great left ventricular pump and thread an artery into it. Now here I was—about to do just that again.

On December 11, 1953, John, sedated, was taken into the operating room. As we expected, there was a huge scar on the front of his heart, and the arteries on the left side of the heart were markedly narrowed and hardened. I probed the chest wall and cautiously teased the left internal mammary artery away from it. The patient's future life depended on an undamaged artery, and, therefore, clamps and forceps could not be used.

I then implanted the artery into healthy muscle beyond the outer side of the scar. From the implanted artery, new vessels would eventually sprout to surrounding tissues. It was a little like the process of planting a tree. You keep some of the earth around

THE OPERATION—STEP 2

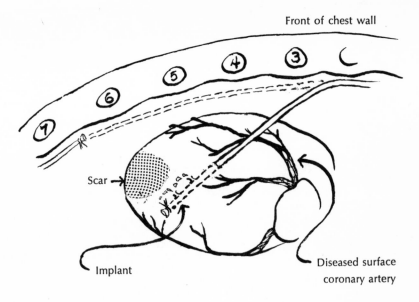

Fig. 4. The left internal mammary artery is implanted in the wall of the left ventricle.

the roots of a small tree that is being transplanted from one location to another, taking care not to damage the roots. Like a tree, the artery must be planted deep in the heart muscle so that it can be properly rooted. And of course, it must enter the muscle without being twisted, coiled, or angled, all of which may block the artery.

I had performed what would later become known around the world as the Vineberg Operation. If successful, blood would, in a few weeks' time, pour through the newly implanted artery into the heart. Six weeks to six months would tell the story. The operation turned out to be a success, and in January 1954, I was quite optimistic about my patient.

"Well, Doc, how do you add it all up?"

John didn't exactly feel he was on top of the world but the pain had subsided. He was about ready to start a new life.

I don't know who was happier about the way it all turned out,

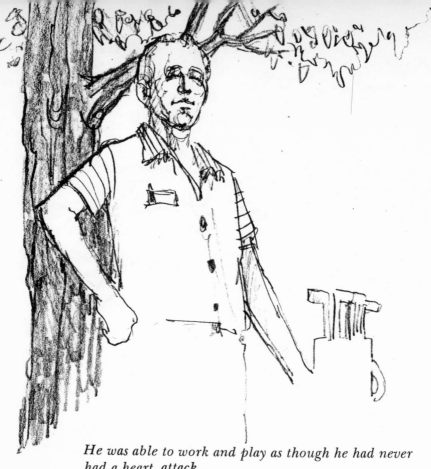

He was able to work and play as though he had never had a heart attack.

John or Catherine. But it was she who kept me posted on things after they had gone home to California.

Among my prize possessions is a Christmas card I received from her in 1954. It reads: "God love you Doctor. John is still working hard. He's big, he's strong—thanks to your kindness and efforts. Will always think of you and thank God you were there."

Every few months, there was a note from Catherine and the news was always good. John was getting better all the time. They finally moved to Nevada and she wrote to say he was now living a completely normal life. He was able to work and play as though he had never had a heart attack.

At Christmas, 1973, Catherine wrote that John was working regularly and thoroughly enjoying life. It was hard to believe. It had been twenty years since I had operated on him.

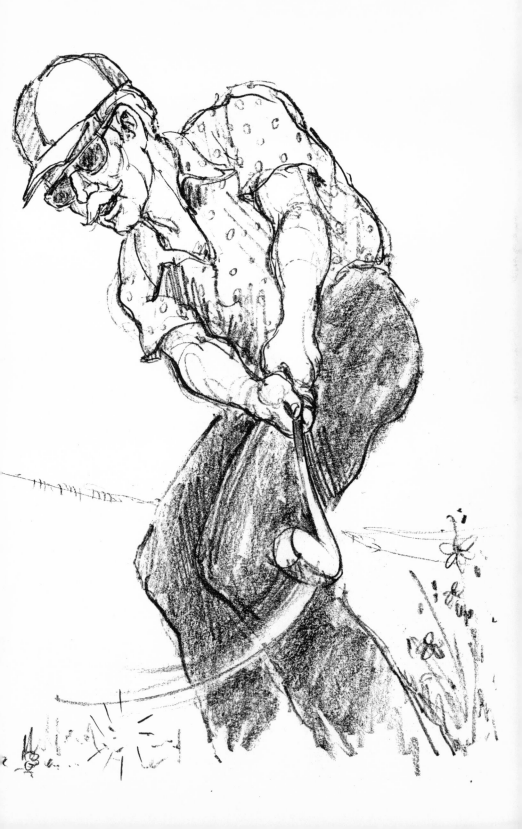

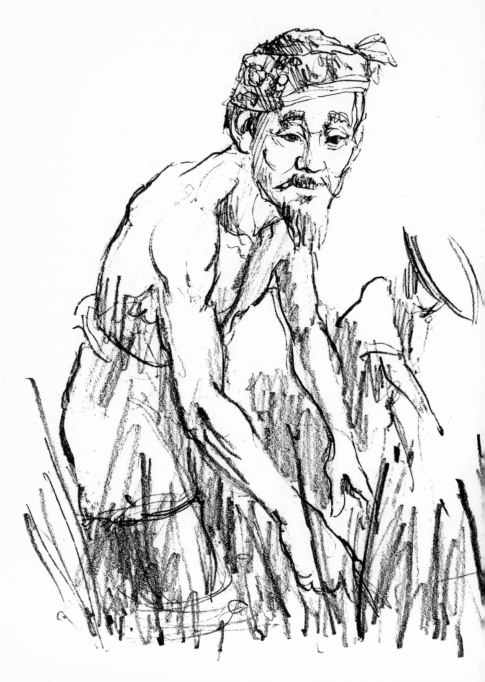

22

Heart Disease in the Western World

Along with cancer, heart disease is the most feared of illnesses. For many, the slightest twinge in the arm or chest suggests an on-coming heart attack. It's not surprising. Practically every time we pick up a newspaper, or turn on the radio, there is news of another heart attack victim. The fact is that coronary artery disease and its complications are presently the major cause of death in America and Western Europe.

The mortality figures are staggering. This year alone some 840,000 people will die from heart disease in the United States and Canada. It is America's biggest killer. It accounts for more than half of all deaths recorded for all diseases, as well as for accidents. It claims almost three times as many lives as does cancer and more than five times the lives lost in accidents.

The statistics tell an interesting story. The annual death rate for coronary artery disease and its complications for all ages and both sexes is 3 per thousand people in the United States and Britain. The rate is 2 per thousand in Denmark, the Netherlands, and Germany, and less than 0.5 per thousand in Japan, China, Ceylon, Central America, and the Indonesian islands.

There is a marked difference between the death rates in afflu-ent Western countries and those in impoverished Eastern countries. Does the way of life of the affluent countries account for it? Are the people of the economically well-to-do countries with their acknowl-edged high standard of living killing themselves with high-fat diets and lack of exercise? There is steadily accumulating evidence to indicate that this is the case. Certainly the figures demand some

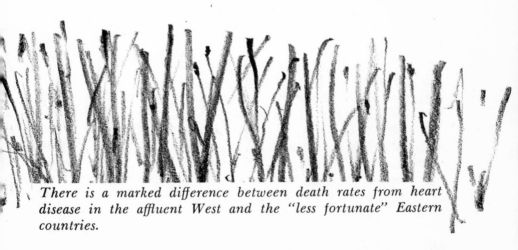

There is a marked difference between death rates from heart disease in the affluent West and the "less fortunate" Eastern countries.

FREQUENCY OF HEART DISEASE AMONG MALES
IN THE UNITED STATES

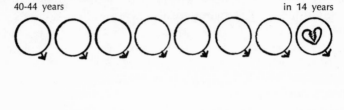

40-44 years   in 14 years

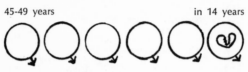

45-49 years   in 14 years

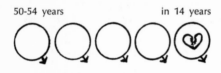

50-54 years   in 14 years

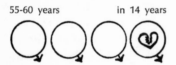

55-60 years   in 14 years

Fig. 5. If you are between 40 and 44 years of age, you have one chance in eight of having a heart attack within 14 years. If you are between 55 and 60 your chances are one in four.

kind of explanation. Consider the category of men 40 to 59 years old; the death rate from coronary disease declines from 8 per thousand in Western countries to less than 1 per thousand in the underprivileged regions of the world.

Although the figures vary from country to country, there has been a significant increase in coronary artery disease over the past 50 years in the Western world. Some astounding early evidence of the extent of the disease came from studies made of Korean war soldiers killed in action. The studies were reported in a 1953 issue of the *Journal of the American Medical Association* by three U.S.

military medical men, Major William F. Enos, Colonel H. Holmes, M.C., and Captain James Beyer, M.C.

Three hundred autopsies of U.S. battle casualties were studied. No one with known clinical evidence of coronary disease was included. The ages of the first 98 men were not recorded. The average age of the last 202, however, was noted—it was 22.1 years, with the oldest man being 48, and the youngest 18 years old. The autopsies showed what the researchers described as "gross evidence" of coronary disease in over 77 percent of the cases. Some of the men had occlusion of one or more major vessels, that is, these blood passageways had become cut off. These were strong, well-nourished, apparently healthy men who at the time of their deaths were physically active and showed no symptomatic evidence of the disease.

On the other hand, the autopsies on Korean soldiers showed only 5 percent with evidence of coronary conditions. East versus West? The figures point up some startling differences in the coronary health of Eastern soldiers and their Western counterparts.

Here are some frightening facts from the well-known Framingham Heart Disease Epidemiology Studies by Drs. T. R. Dawber, W. B. Kannel, and W. P. Castelli: They studied the frequency of coronary artery heart disease in a large group of people living in and about Framingham, Massachusetts over an 18-year period. From this they concluded that in the United States of America every eighth male now between 40 and 44 years of age will have a heart attack within 14 years. Every sixth man now between 45 and 49 will have an attack within 14 years. Every fifth man over the age of 50 and every fourth between 55 and 60 will have an attack within 14 years. By the age of 60, every fifth male will have had a heart attack.

More frightening still is the fact that the average age of the heart attack victim is becoming younger. It is no longer unusual for a man to have an attack before he is 40.

The figures are alarming. Even more shocking is the certain knowledge that so many of these attacks and deaths are unnecessary.

Unnecessary for two reasons: first, in a great number of cases, heart disease *can* be prevented; second, all heart attack victims do not have to live out their lives as cardiac cripples.

We have amassed a great deal of information about the heart. We know a lot about prevention. In surgery, we have made tremendous strides toward the conquest of coronary artery heart disease. Yet, over the years the statistics have shown a steady increase in incidence of heart disease. What is the explanation?

Despite the progress that has been made, we are still lacking adequate instruments to detect developing conditions. It is a staggering fact that 20–30 percent of all electrocardiograms are inaccurate. Many a man has died minutes after being told he has a clear cardiogram.

Not only are we not diagnosing correctly in many cases—frequently we give ineffective treatment in cases where a proper diagnosis has been made.

For years, the treatment of angina pectoris (pain in the pectoral or nipple area) due to coronary artery disease has been almost entirely medical (as opposed to surgical). Doctors gave their patients certain drugs, told them to rest up, but often, could do nothing more than sit placidly and watch the patients die. For many years, this was accepted treatment; regrettably it is still the way many heart patients are looked after. Moreover, reports of successful treatment by such medical measures must now be seri-

All heart attack victims do not have to live out their lives as cardiac cripples.

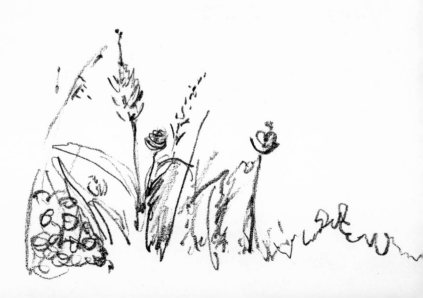

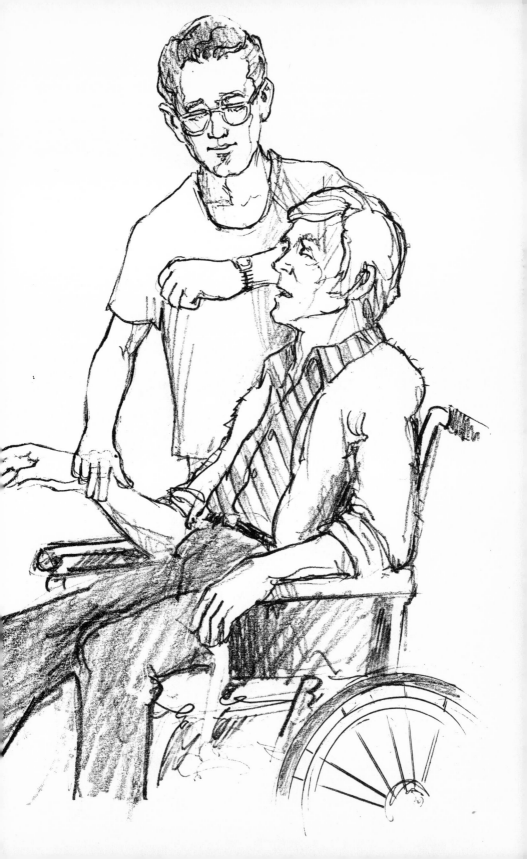

TRIPLE AORTO-CORONARY VEIN
BYPASS OPERATION

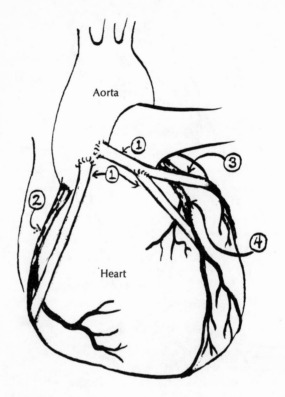

Fig. 6. (1) Vein bypass.
      (2) Diseased right coronary artery.
      (3) Diseased circumflex coronary artery.
      (4) Diseased anterior descending coronary artery.

ously questioned, since the coronary arteries of the individuals concerned had not been examined by modern scientific means.

At present there are no *medical* measures that have been proven to stop the progress of hardening of the arteries, and certainly none that are known to reverse it. I challenge anyone to refute this statement.

Medical treatment with drugs may help some patients symptomatically for a time. However, all medical measures known to us today are palliative. For example, there is no evidence that a narrowed coronary artery becomes widened again, or that a fully obstructed artery reopens through medical treatment.

Cases of heart failure can be controlled with diuretics (drugs that remove excess fluid from the body) and such stimulants as digitalis. There are dilating drugs that are administered to open up the arteries, and other drugs that lower the blood pressure, thus reducing the strain on the heart. But patients who take these drugs are never *cured*. They have to continue taking drugs—and always, their treatment is only palliative. What is needed are means of preventing atherosclerosis, but even if these means are found, the hardened obstructive coronary arteries now present will not change.

The answer then for many is surgery—but here we are faced with the dilemma of the cardiologist who doesn't share this view.

It is a fact that many doctors do not refer their patients to surgeons. Or they will refer the patient only as a last resort—when he can no longer work, or when he has wound up as an emergency case in a hospital coronary care unit.

Some younger cardiologists will suggest consultation with a surgeon. Still, probably no more than 25,000 coronary operations are performed a year in America. This is a very small figure when you consider that over 800,000 people die during the same period. Right now, there are probably some 500,000 people in the United States and Canada who could benefit from surgery. The vast majority, however, will never reach an operating room, often because of the reluctance of their doctors. There are many centers where various types of revascularization operations are done, but cardiologist resistance is still strong.

Many centers perform the aorto-coronary vein bypass operation, but this covers less than one-tenth of the number needed. The Vineberg Operation is also being performed, either alone or in combination with aorto-coronary vein bypass grafts, in many Canadian and American cities. (Fig. 6.) (See chapters on Surgery.)

29

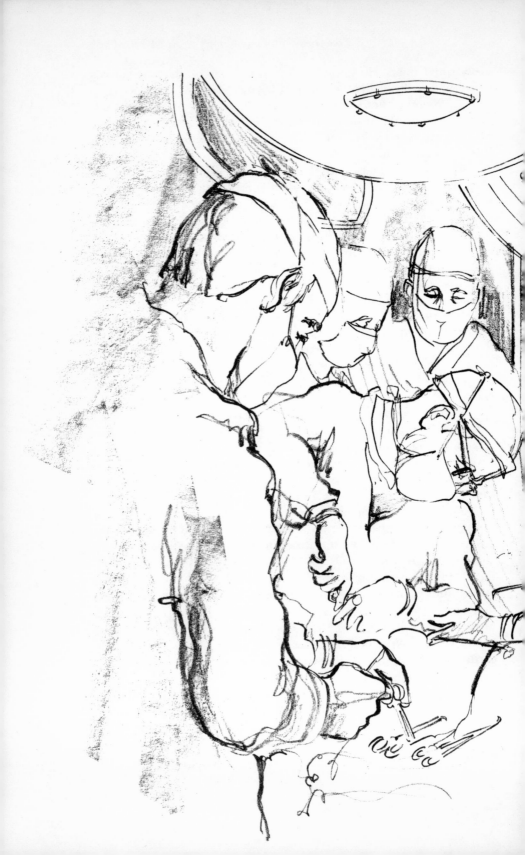

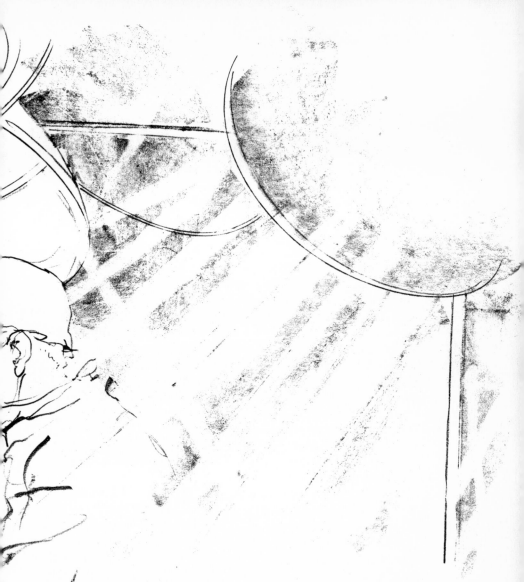

I am not suggesting that everyone who has a heart attack should have surgery. Thousands of autopsies show evidence of two or three heart attacks which went unknown to the person or his doctors. The person may have simply felt tired or thought he had indigestion, never suspecting that something was wrong with his heart.

Any person suffering from proven coronary artery disease, whose symptoms persist more than six months, should have his arteries studied to determine the seriousness of the disease. If the symptoms are still there at the end of a year, surgery may be indicated.

The success rate of our revascularization procedures is high. It has a less than 2 percent operative loss. That is, less than 2 percent of patients die within thirty days of the operation. Even in extremely advanced cases, the loss is under 10 percent. Eighty-five percent of those who have revascularization live more than five and a half years after their operations, and many live twelve to twenty years after. Thus, many will live out their normal span of years as if they never had the disease.

I am often asked how many of the 840,000 people who die annually of heart disease could be saved by surgery. It's not an easy question because a great many factors are involved. But on the basis of a recent study of autopsy records, I am able to offer a projection.

According to pathological studies, less than 3 percent of the coronary cases that ended up in the autopsy room were in the inoperable category before death. The other 97 percent had at least half of their heart muscle left. Now, if a new supply of blood could have been introduced into the still healthy part of the muscle, I believe most of them could have been saved.

If we can get blood into the healthy muscle, we can give the patient great help. He may not be able to do the hundred yard dash, but he will be able to live without pain and earn a living for his family.

At this very moment, millions of young men are on a coronary collision course which, if unchecked, will kill them or maim them in the prime of their lives. I want to reach them before it is too late.

I want to reach the others, too, the staggering number of individuals who have already experienced a coronary attack. I want to tell them that all is not lost, that indeed there is hope.

I want to tell the mothers of young children and the wives of the coronary-prone how they can go about safeguarding their men. The women are the ones who can really do this job because, in the final analysis, they are the most health-conscious. Call it vanity, or any other name, but in their desire to be attractive, they make a much greater effort to look after their bodies than do men.

Women count the calories they eat, and they exercise. You'll find them in the gymnasium, on the tennis courts, in reducing classes, and in yoga classes, learning breathing exercises. You'll also find them doing rigorous exercise at home in the normal, day-to-day business of running a house. If any man doubts the exercise factor in housework, let him try making a bed.

There is no magic formula for the elimination of heart disease.

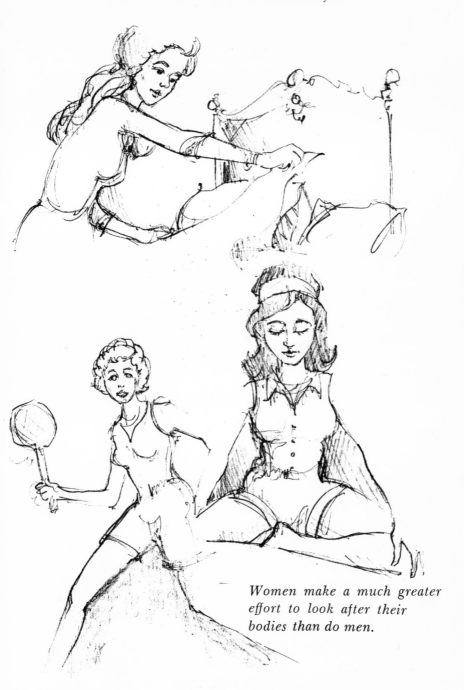

Women make a much greater effort to look after their bodies than do men.

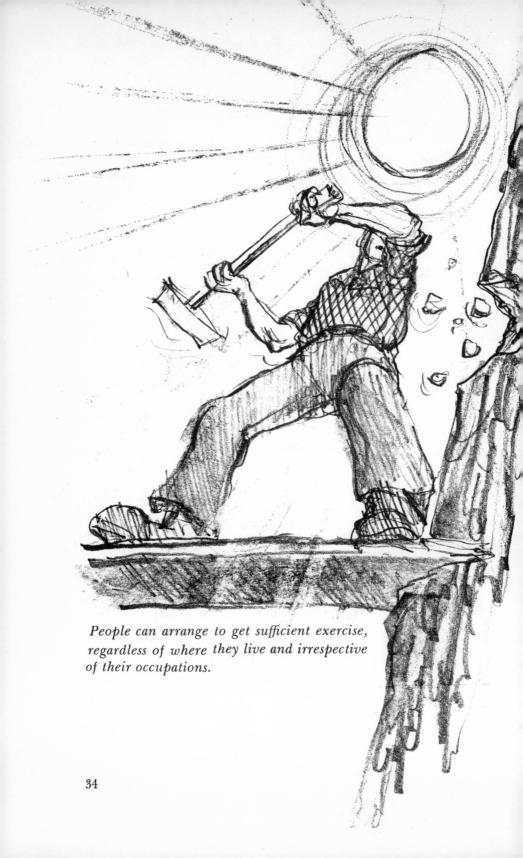

*People can arrange to get sufficient exercise,
regardless of where they live and irrespective
of their occupations.*

34

You can't take a pill to make you immune. But millions of people could avoid the disease by following certain basic rules of good health. Easy as it may sound, though, this is not simple advice to follow.

We hear a lot about the hazards of over-eating and of smoking. We're constantly reminded that we don't do nearly enough exercise. Leave the car at home and walk, we're urged. But let me ask you. When did you last keep a cholesterol-conscious diet? Have you given up smoking? When did you last leave the car at home and walk?

People can't help inheriting heart disease, nor can they always avoid tension-producing situations. But they *can* watch their food intake.

In the appendix to this book, there is an extensive list of foods. The tables are designed for quick, easy reference. They give you not only the calorie count of various foods, they also list the cholesterol count. They can show you how to eat well and still control your calorie and cholesterol intake.

People *can* also arrange to get sufficient exercise, regardless of whether they live in the city or in the country, and irrespective of their occupations. I won't suggest a rigorous program of jogging because contrary to what many people think, severe jogging can be dangerous. In fact, it can kill you. But regular exercise is necessary and you can find the activity that best suits your needs by checking the exercise tables in this book. They spell out the amount of energy required to perform each activity.

As you read this book, you will understand why I don't believe in the absolute inevitability of heart disease. But I am a realist— and I know it will not be easy to follow my advice. Yet, if the young are to reach old age with their hearts healthy and pumping vigorously, then the advice in this book must be heeded.

Finally, I shall make no extravagant claims. I shall simply show that heart disease is often preventable and that there is high hope for those already afflicted with the disease.

CHAPTER 2

Your Heart—How It Works

The human heart is a wonderful machine, regulating the flow of blood over an incredible 100,000 miles of pipeline—the blood vessels.

It is roughly the size of a clenched fist, some 5 inches long, $3\frac{1}{2}$ inches wide and about half an inch thick. It is a power plant that weighs 11 ounces in a man and only 9 in a woman; yet, it operates a blood vessel network which, measured in miles, is more than four times the distance around the circumference of the earth.

The heart is the measure of life. Its beat marks the beginning and the end. To understand it is to understand the mechanism of life.

THE FOUR CHAMBER HEART

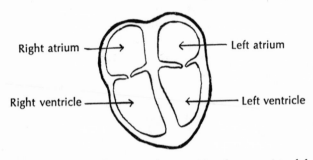

Fig. 7. The human heart can be considered to consist of four separate pumps.

The heart is divided into four chambers. The two upper chambers, the *atria,* or *auricles,* collect the blood flowing into the heart. The lower chambers, the *ventricles,* pump blood into the arteries. The right ventricle sends blood to the lungs. The left sends blood throughout the body.

The four-chamber heart is present in most animals as well as in humans. In primitive creatures such as the jelly-fish there is no heart. Circulation is by diffusion. In the lower animals there is a single chamber representing one pump. The human heart, however, can be considered as being composed of four separate pumps. (Fig. 7).

The wall of each pump is made up of heart muscle, which is very different from the skeletal muscle that moves arms, legs, and other parts of the body. While the latter contract only when motion is necessary, the heart pump muscle contracts continuously. They start early in the pregnancy and continue day and night until we die.

The heart pumps blood to other parts of the body but it too must receive nourishment and here the great life-giving currents go into reverse. Blood flows to the heart muscles through the coronary arteries that lie over the walls of the heart. These are divided into smaller and smaller arteries that branch and dip into the heart muscle ending in separate arteriolar zones.

The coronary arteries make up an intricate and fascinating map. I think of them as forming an arterial tree. The situation here can be compared to an irrigation system supplying fresh water to an area through two large conduits (right and left coronary arteries) which leave a large body of water (aorta) through the wall of a dam. (Fig. 8). The left divides into two coronary arteries (called anterior descending and circumflex). The three divide into smaller pipelines (smaller surface arteries) feeding water into small canals (myocardial arterioles).

Each major pipeline system supplies its own territory and each coronary artery does the same. (Fig. 8). If one pipeline is narrowed, the area which it irrigates does not receive sufficient water and the trees and vegetation wither and die. When disease occurs in the coronary arterial tree, it is disseminated, thus narrowing not only the major pipelines but many of the branches on the surface of the heart. It does not, however, involve the canals which actually do the irrigation, delivering the water to the soil. These canals can be compared to the myocardial arteriolar networks and they never become blocked except in patients with severe diabetes and long-standing high blood pressure.

This is the reason for revascularization surgery. Internal mammary arteries are implanted into the walls of the right and left great pumps where the nondiseased arteriolar vessels lie. This is the same as laying a new pipeline in the soil. (Fig. 9). Rusty pipelines in the earth are difficult to repair, and unblocking them is not a permanent solution. You really need new rust-resistant copper piping. The same goes for coronary arteries. New pipelines are needed here which don't become diseasesd. Internal mammary arteries are ideal in this respect.

In most human hearts, the canals supplied by one coronary artery are separated from the canals supplied by another. (Fig. 8). In order to bring water to a dry area, the gates between adjoining canals (myocardial arteriolar networks) have to be opened to allow water to flow from one area to another.

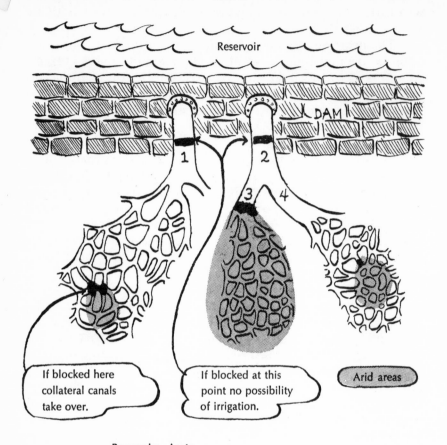

Reservoir

DAM

1

2

3   4

If blocked here
collateral canals
take over.

If blocked at this
point no possibility
of irrigation.

Arid areas

Reservoir: Aorta

Conduit 1: Right coronary artery

Conduit 2: Left coronary artery

Conduit 3: Anterior descending coronary artery

Conduit 4: Circumflex coronary artery

Fig. 8. Think of the coronary arterial system as a series of pipelines, remembering that the problems that occur in an industrial
pipeline can also happen in the human system.

The coronary arterial system is not too difficult to understand
if one thinks of it as a series of pipelines. The fact is that the problems that occur in an industrial pipeline also happen in the coronary system. What damages a commercial line will also hurt the
body's pipelines.

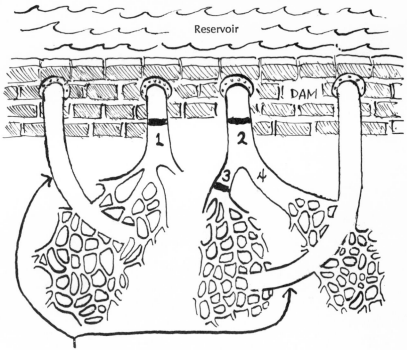

Non-diseased internal mammary arteries

Reservoir: Aorta

Conduit 1: Right coronary artery

Conduit 2: Left coronary artery

Conduit 3: Anterior descending coronary artery

Conduit 4: Circumflex coronary artery

Fig. 9. Implanted internal mammary arteries allow oxygenated blood to flow into the "arid" areas.

We shall explore the probable causes of coronary artery disease later, but for the moment we may assume that the end result is the same. Simply stated, there is a reduction in oxygenated blood for the hard-working heart plant.

So much for blackboard explanations. Now let us examine heart conditions from the patient's point of view.

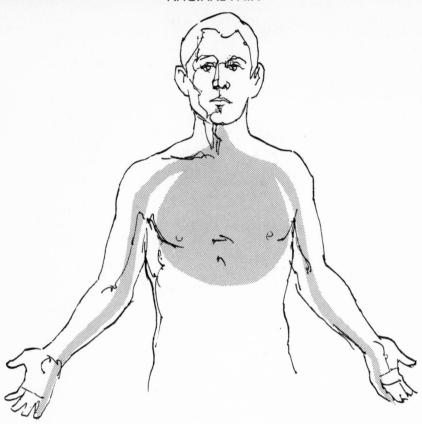

Fig. 10. The distribution of anginal pain is depicted by shaded areas.

Angina Pectoris

Angina pectoris is a term that has almost become a household word in recent years. It means pain in the pectoral, or nipple region. (Fig. 10). The pain may originate from many causes, but it has been linked most frequently with the narrowing of a coronary artery. It is a warning signal to the brain that the heart muscle is not getting enough oxygenated blood to allow it to work properly.

Pain may be felt in the region of the nipples but it may also be felt in the center of the chest. It may go down the left arm or both arms, up to the neck and even down into the abdomen. It may be very short-lived and go away when the stimulating cause has been removed.

In some cases, the pain is quite severe. One patient told me it was as though an elephant had been sitting on his chest. Another said his chest felt as though it were in a vice. The pain may not recur for some days, and it may not come back for some years for that matter. After experiencing any such pain, however, it is vital that a cardiologist be consulted.

True anginal pain is due to the fact that an insufficient amount of oxygenated blood reaches the left ventricular pump muscle, and even perhaps the right ventricular heart muscle. It is not surprising then that as the artery supplying the muscle of the contracting heart wall becomes progressively narrowed, it takes less effort and excitement to bring on pain. When all three coronary arteries become narrowed, so little oxygenated blood reaches the heart muscle that the heart can no longer pump effectively.

In very advanced cases, the heart machine reaches a point where it hasn't enough oxygenated blood to maintain minimum circulation without pain even when a patient is at rest in a chair or in bed. I think of this situation in terms of a red light, flashing sometimes up to 40 times in a 24-hour period, to indicate an empty fuel tank for the heart muscle pump.

The state in which the act of lying at rest produces anginal pain is known as *angina decubitus,* that is, angina pectoris at rest without exciting cause.

When part of the heart muscle receives no blood because of complete blockage of a coronary artery the area becomes arid. In a land irrigation system, living matter dies if the acreage is deprived of water due to a blocked pipeline. (Fig. 8). When an area of heart muscle has no irrigation by oxygenated blood because of a blocked, or markedly narrowed, coronary artery, the heart muscle stops contracting and dies. The patient may die after the heart stops but if only part of the heart muscle is affected, it may continue to beat and the patient experiences a *myocardial infarction,* or heart attack.

A severe heart attack is usually signaled by almost unbearable squeezing pain in the center of the chest. Unlike previous anginal pectoris pains, it doesn't disappear, and persists even if the excitement or activity which caused it is gone. Usually the patient is cold, clammy, weak, and sweaty. Furthermore, unlike the other anginal pains the patient has experienced, this pain is not relieved by drugs such as nitroglycerine and may require many injections of morphine. The doctor is need immediately and hospitalization in a coronary care unit is the next move. The pain may last anywhere from an hour to a few days.

Death from the first heart attack occurs in approximately 15 percent of cases. For some of the remaining 85 percent, recovery may be complete with the patient experiencing no heart pain, that is no anginal pain, for a number of years. There may be no symptoms involving the heart and the subject may be able to carry on a normal, active life. More likely, however, recovery will not be complete. In fact, pain may occur more frequently than before the heart attack and exercise and work may be more difficult to perform.

After one heart attack, there is a 15 percent chance of dying for each year of life. After a second heart attack, 18 to 20 percent of patients may die per year. After a third attack, the prospects are gloomy indeed. Of 100 patients, most would be dead within five years if they continued to suffer anginal pain.

We must differentiate between people who have heart attacks which are not followed by anginal pain, and those who have attacks and continue to have pain, sometimes even more severe than previously.

In the first group, an area of the heart muscle dies, together with the nerve endings within it. The dead heart muscle then is replaced by scars which do not contain nerve endings. Patients may have no pain if surrounding arteries provide enough oxygenated blood to the remaining heart muscle.

In the second group, in which the pain persists or becomes worse after an attack, the remaining heart muscle is not receiving enough oxygenated blood to keep it functioning properly without sending distress signals to the brain. It is more and more difficult for such hearts, having lost between 20 and 30 percent of their muscle, to carry on the pumping action necessary for a normal life.

The normal heart pump pushes the blood out into the *aorta* (the largest blood vessel coming from the heart and the center from which the arterial system proceeds) (Fig. 1) at the rate of at least 6.5 quarts per minute. This is known as the cardiac output. This fresh oxygenated blood reaches every part of the body, delivering nourishing sugars, proteins, fats, salts, and oxygen to every living cell. To pump effectively, the muscular wall of the left ventricular pump must be healthy. After an attack, part of the heart muscle dies and is replaced by scar. During healing, there is a soft, bulging spot—which does not contract—in the wall of the left ventricular pump.

If this is extensive, the damaged left pump may not be able to push out all the oxygenated blood sent to it and a backing-up occurs. Fluids are retained in the lungs, making them stiff and unable to exchange gases, a condition leading to poor oxygenation.

When the right ventricular pump also fails, fluids are retained in the abdomen and legs as well and they likewise become swollen.

When this happens, we have what is commonly known as heart failure.

Heart failure is a condition that may develop without myocardial infarction, that is without a heart attack, when the heart muscle, though still alive, is terribly weak due to a poor supply of oxygenated blood. This occurs when the arteries are so greatly narrowed that the muscular wall of the left ventricular pump obtains insufficient fuel. It does not die but it keeps contracting so poorly, it cannot push out enough oxygenated blood to maintain body health. There is an inevitable backup with a resulting retention of fluid in the lungs, abdomen and legs.

We have learned a lot about this intricate machine we call the heart. But are we simply well-informed in an academic sense, or are we able to make use of our extensive knowledge in a practical way? What about diagnosis? How good are modern methods of detection? Are doctors able to recognize and identify the causes of heart pain?

Let us examine the situation.

CHAPTER 3

Diagnosis — The Heart Attack

A heart attack can strike with devastating swiftness, crippling the victim and sometimes killing him. It can also come upon him slowly, with considerable advance warning, giving time to get help before it's too late.

Many of the aches and pains of everyday life are muscular in origin, the result of a sudden twist, or wrench, or just plain over-exertion. But some are not—and your familiarity with the danger signs might just mean the difference between life and death.

Stated simply:

Any pain in the center of the chest, anywhere along the breast plate, around the nipples, or in the left arm, shoulder or neck, could be a warning signal.

If the pain occurs during a period of emotion or excitement, then quickly disappears after the period is over, make mental note of the experience.

If the pain recurs under similar circumstances at a later date, see a doctor because you could be headed for a heart attack.

The same advice applies if you get pain during exercise, such as walking up stairs, for example.

The first pain is a routine warning. The second, occurring under the same conditions, is a flashing red signal. It is the repetition of the pain that is the urgent warning.

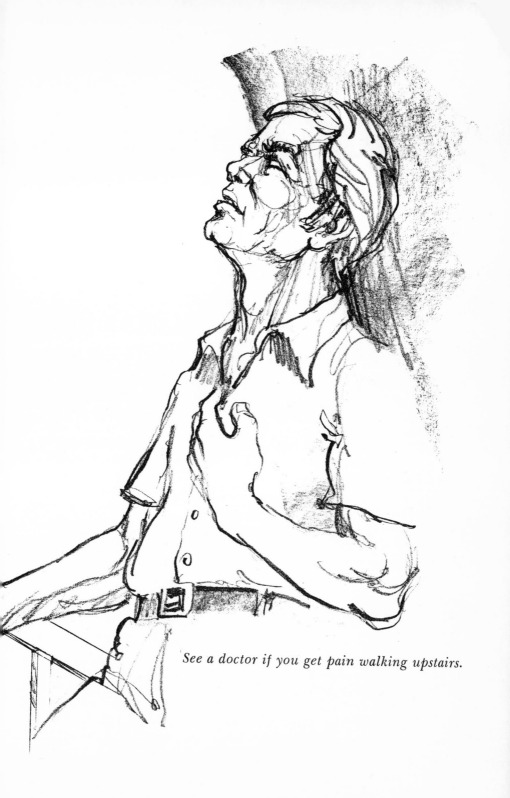

See a doctor if you get pain walking upstairs.

The early warning pains may not be too well-defined at first—but if you are actually having a heart attack, chances are you will soon realize it.

The pain will most likely be severe, even crushing.

Usually, it strikes in the center of the chest—but sometimes it occurs in the lower part of the chest, or in the arms. (Fig. 10).

It may feel like a fist, crashing relentlessly through the chest wall. Or like a metal band being pulled ever so tightly around the chest.

It will be difficult to take a deep breath, usually, in fact, it is not possible.

The hands become cold and clammy.

The forehead is covered with sweat—often *cold* sweat.

The face becomes gray in color.

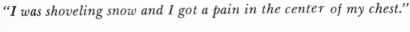

"I was shoveling snow and I got a pain in the center of my chest."

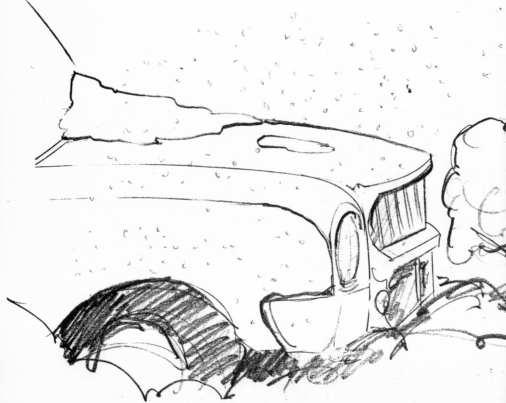

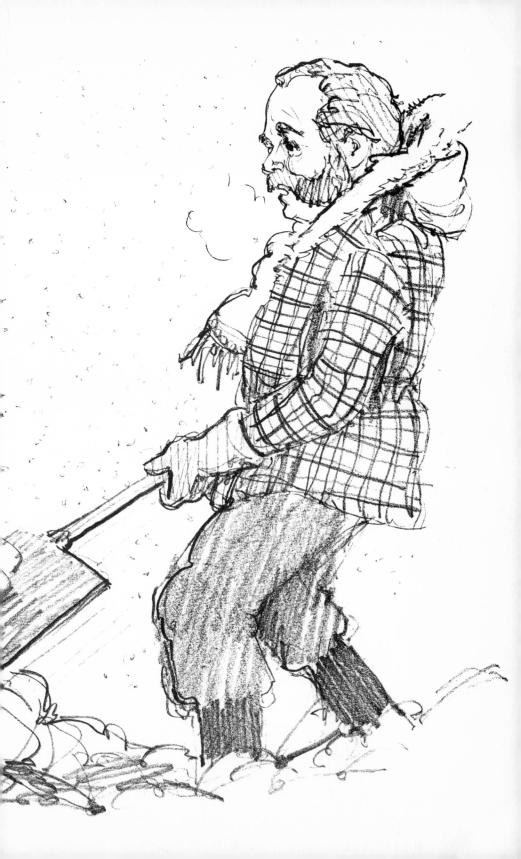

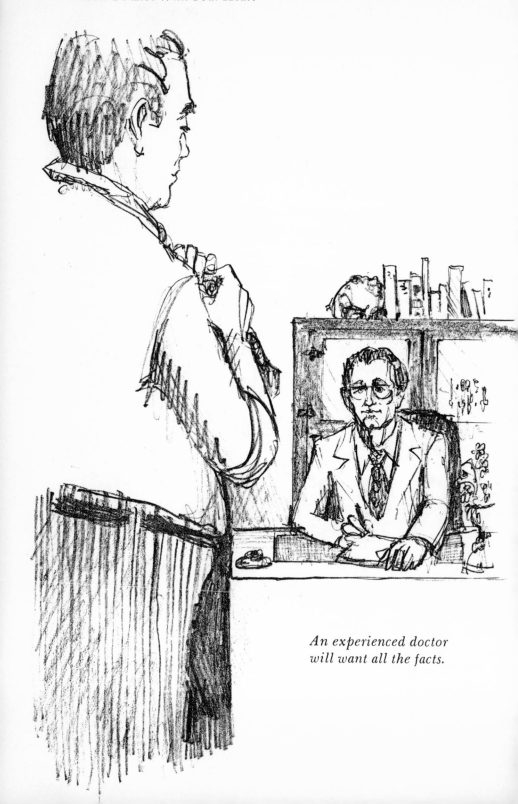

*An experienced doctor
will want all the facts.*

The pain itself could indicate a gallbladder attack, or a bout of indigestion. However, if you sweat, it's almost certainly a heart attack. You don't sweat with gallbladder trouble, nor with indigestion.

Upon having these symptoms, lie flat down, or propped up by pillows, whichever position makes you more comfortable.

Stay as quiet as you can for half an hour. If the pain persists, call a doctor, or a hospital. Failing that, call the police.

I address this advice to the person who is having his first attack —but it applies as well to the individual with a previous history of anginal pain.

If you are in the latter category, I have this advice:

If you have taken medication in the past, do so again. Nitroglycerine tablets might help; if they do not, get to the hospital as quickly as you can.

Recognizing The Symptoms

Recognizing the symptoms of a heart attack could some day save your life. Being able to describe them will help the doctor diagnose your case with accuracy.

Despite the development of sophisticated equipment, the most important single method of diagnosis of anginal pain caused by diseased coronary arteries still rests in the description given by the patient of his or her chest pain. A wise physician and cardiologist do well to spend an hour or more questioning the patient about the pain. It is most important to get the history of the pain from the very first time the patient had been aware of it.

The experienced doctor wants all the facts and his questioning can be very exhaustive, as the following case report indicates:

"When were you last perfectly well?" the cardiologist asks.
"About four years ago," the patient replies.
"What happened then?"
"I was shoveling snow and I got a pain in the center of my chest."
"Did you stop shoveling?"
"Yes."
"Did the pain go away?"
"It did."
"Did you have the pain again?"
"Yes, two years later. I ran for a bus and it was a cold day and suddenly I had the pain again."
"When did you have a pain that didn't go away?"

49

"A year or so ago. It came just after dinner and lasted all night."
"Did you sweat?"
"Yes."
"Did you call a doctor?"
"Yes. He said I had had a heart attack and sent me to hospital."
"How long were you off work?"
"About three months."
"Do you have the pain now?"
"Yes."
"When does it come?"

The pain varies a great deal from patient to patient and even varies from time to time in the same individual. Thus, the answers to this question are often different.

"When I get up in the morning," one person says.
"After breakfast," a second states.
"When I go to get the car out of the garage," someone explains.

The patient's answers determine the course of subsequent questioning.

"I don't have any pain until I get to work," one man points out.
"What brings on the pain there?" the doctor inquires.
"Different things. I get pain sometimes when I get angry. Or if I have a long telephone conversation, or if I'm involved in a lengthy conference. Just picking up something heavy will do it on occasion."
"Do drugs help?"
"Nitroglycerine relieves the pain."
"How long does it take?"
"Three or four minutes."

There are many variations to contend with. Some patients, for example, have no chest pains preceding a heart attack. Others have *silent heart attacks,* in which case there is no pain signal to warn the patient that he is having an attack.

For most patients, anginal pain follows a pattern. It is usually felt in the center of the chest, is squeezing or pressing in type, goes across the pectoral regions and may go down the left arm or both

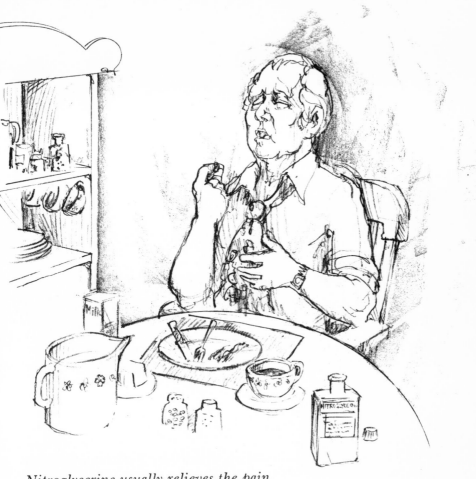

Nitroglycerine usually relieves the pain.

arms. In some cases it goes up into the neck and in others through the chest to the back between the shoulder blades. It is brought on, among other things, by excitement, effort, walking into a wind, and after eating. It disappears when the cause is removed, lasting usually not longer than a few minutes.

There is a variation in frequency of attacks among patients. An individual may have none for two weeks and then have two or three daily. It is not unusual for an attack to produce a burning sensation often mistaken for indigestion.

A typical interview might continue as follows:

"How far can you walk on the street, keeping up with the speed of the crowd?"
"About two blocks."
"Then what?"
"Because I have pain I stop and window-shop."
"Does it go away with nitroglycerine?"
"Yes."
"Do you use more than one pillow at night?"
"I use three."
"Three? Why?"
"Because I get shortness of breath and pain in my chest."
"Do you have a large breakfast?"
"Yes, often. When I do I get pain walking to the car."
"Were your legs swollen at any time?"
"They were some time ago. They aren't now."
"What happened?"
"My doctor gave me pills to get rid of the fluid."

This is important evidence. A person who retains excessive amounts of fluid may well be suffering a degree of heart failure.

"You say when you walk on the street you have to stop because you have shortness of breath. Do you mean that you pant like a dog running?"
"No. I can't get my breath because of a tightness in my chest."
"If you walk on a cold day or in the wind, do you get the pain?"
"Yes."

The patient's description of his discomfort tells much about his condition. That "tightness in the chest" suggests an arterial problem rather than a simple situation of being *out of breath.* The fact that he gets pain walking is another indication of a heart problem. Pain that comes without exercise or excitement is not likely related to a coronary condition. It may result from diseases of the gallbladder, from hiatus hernia (when part of the stomach slides up into the chest), or from diseased discs in the neck.

The Hereditary Factor

Coronary artery disease, like diabetes, tends to run in families, so a doctor does well to look closely at his patient's family tree.

One of the patients I have treated can serve as an example. He is a doctor in Tampa, Florida, and a former football player,

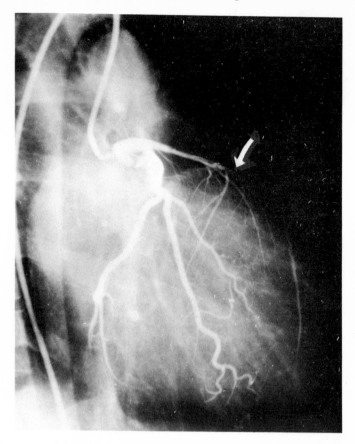

CINE CORONARY ARTERIOGRAPHY

Fig. 11. Reproduction from an arteriogram of a diseased left coronary artery, showing its irregularities and areas of obstruction.

who came to see me after recovering from a heart attack. He had no pain. What worried him was that he had three brothers with anginal pain.

We examined him through a Cine Coronary Anteriogram (see Dictionary) and found that all three coronary arteries were diseased. He had no symptoms. However, I recommended surgery. The patient, a doctor himself, was content to leave things as they were and returned to Florida. Then one day, he telephoned me:

"How soon can you arrange an operation?" he wanted to know.

"What's the hurry?" I asked.

"I told you about my three brothers having anginal pain.

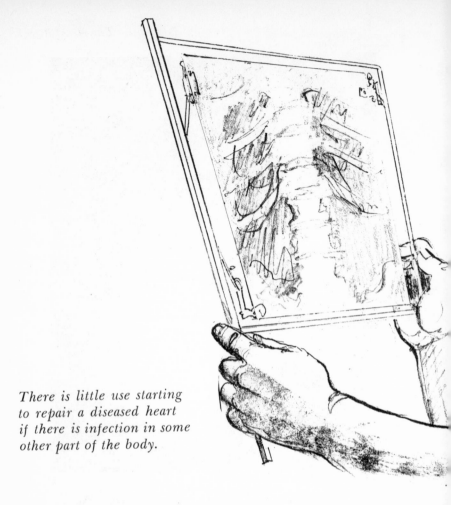

*There is little use starting
to repair a diseased heart
if there is infection in some
other part of the body.*

Well, two of them have died since I saw you. And the third is right
now in hospital with a heart attack."

The doctor from Tampa got his wish. I operated on him. He
was the only patient without symptoms I had ever taken into surgery—and he still is. I operated on him solely on the basis of his
family history and, of course, the extent of the coronary artery
occlusions shown by Cine Coronary Arteriography.

Family history is very relevant. I want to know about a man's
brothers and sisters, about his parents and grandparents. I want to
know who had a heart condition and who died from it.

I look, too, for a history of elevated blood cholesterol, and
triglycerides, a condition caused by a person's inability to handle
blood fats found in certain foods. Most doctors agree that elevated
blood cholesterol and triglyceride levels also tend to run in families.
Thus when such a history is present, pain in the pectoral area must

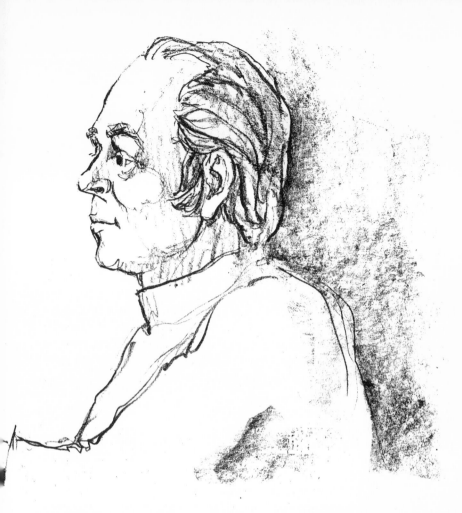

be considered as a possible result of trouble in the coronary arteries.

Now a word of caution: people with no family history of coronary artery disease must not conclude that they are immune, that they cannot get the disease. A person cannot hide behind a good inheritance. Even the strongest machine can break down through misuse or abuse.

There are other conditions frequently associated with coronary disease. For example, there is a tendency for patients with persistently high blood pressure and diabetes to develop *atherosclerosis,* particularly involving the coronary arteries. Atherosclerosis is a condition of both softening and hardening of the artery wall. It leads to narrowing—and sometimes blocking—of the artery.

The discovery of diseased arteries elsewhere in the body, such as the legs, resulting in cramps in the calves after walking a short distance, or the finding of disease in one of the vessels of the neck which causes dizziness, is evidence of possible coronary atherosclerosis. The disease may also strike certain young women who have had hysterectomies. The ovaries are often removed with the womb resulting in cessation of estrogen production. Estrogen is said to protect the female from coronary artery disease.

Throughout my practice, I have believed in treating the whole patient and not just part of him. There is little use starting to repair a diseased heart if there is infection in some other part of the body. Any infection that exists should be cleared up before surgery. For this reason, every patient who comes to me is put through a series of routine examinations.

The sinuses, teeth, urinary and genital tracts are checked. Routine X rays are taken of the chest, stomach, gallbladder, and large bowel. The heart is examined for size, contractility, and the presence of *aneurysms* (weak spots in the walls of the ventricle). Extensive blood chemistry studies are made, particularly if a patient has been on *diuretics,* the fluid-removing pills. Studies are concerned among other things with the heart's clotting mechanism. The blood may have a tendency of clotting rapidly, thus confronting the patient with an added hazard.

The Electrocardiogram

In addition to the examinations and inquiries, an electrocardiogram is taken. It is compared, where possible, with any previous ones that may have been taken over the years.

The electrocardiogram, misunderstood by so many, is really a simple process. It registers electrical current set up by contracting heart muscle. Areas of the muscle that contract badly due to a poor blood supply, or because of a scar from an earlier heart attack, may be detected through a change in the electrical activity of these areas.

How effective is the electrocardiogram at finding trouble spots in the heart?

The value of the electrocardiogram should not be negated. It has been extremely useful in a great many instances. In fact, many people may well owe their lives to the technique, as its warning signal enabled them to get medical help while there was still time.

But there is another side to the matter and this must be clearly understood. Sometimes there are errors. Every doctor has at one time or another come across an erroneous ECG (electrocardiogram) which is normal even when there is extensive coronary artery disease present. And many a family has been shocked by a father's

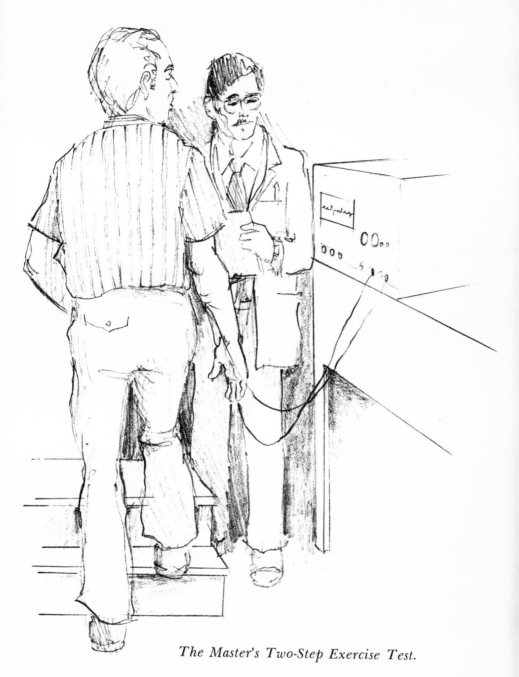

The Master's Two-Step Exercise Test.

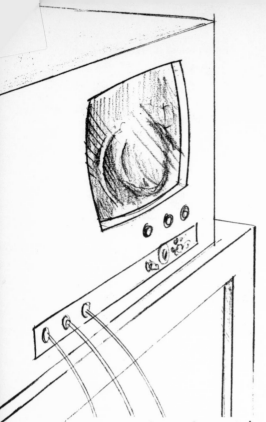

The most important test is the Cine Coronary Arteriography procedure.

fatal heart attack shortly after an electrocardiogram has given him a clean bill of health. It is a distressing matter of record that the ECG all too frequently appears normal in the presence of a dangerous coronary artery condition.

The element of error hardly can be ignored when one considers that ECGs are inaccurate in 20 to 30 percent of cases. Pity the poor patient whose doctor is basing his diagnosis on evidence with such a margin of error.

Inaccuracies occur in electrocardiograms taken both when the patient is at rest and also exercising. For the latter ECGs, patients may be given the *Master's Two-Step Exercise Test* if their ECGs are normal at rest. This requires the patient to go up and down two steps a number of times, depending upon age and weight. The test is safe when conducted under expert supervision. It should under no circumstances be undertaken if there is evidence of an impending heart attack. Many centers exercise patients on a treadmill instead of the Master's test, recording heart action by an electrocardiogram during the exercise.

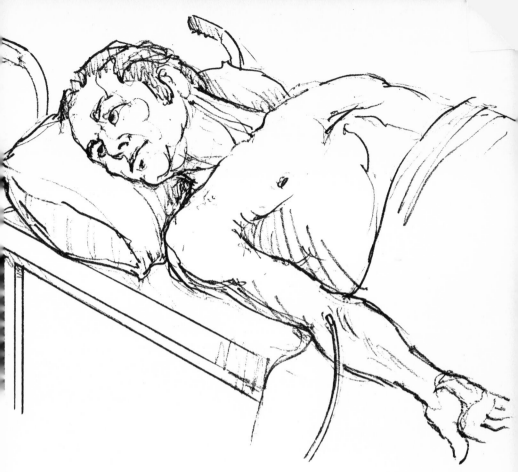

Cine Coronary Arteriography

Because of the electrocardiogram's less-than-perfect performance history, I do not rely on this particular method of diagnosis alone—and neither should your doctor.

Fortunately, other tests have been devised. The most important of these is a remarkable procedure called *Cine Coronary Arteriography,* which provides a motion picture record of what goes on in the coronary system. This picture is known as a coronary arteriogram.

For this test, the patient goes to a laboratory. He lies on a table and a small tube is guided into the mouth of the left coronary artery through an artery in the leg or arm. Into this tube a small amount of solution which shows on an X ray is injected into the coronary artery and its passage down the coronary arterial trunk and its branches is followed by an *image intensifier,* a highly complex camera which makes a moving picture record of the entire procedure.

After the left coronary artery has been examined, the tube is then pushed along the aorta into the chamber of the left ventricle to record the pressures within it. More solution is injected. This outlines the walls of the left ventricular pump, showing areas which are not contracting either because they are *ischemic* (lacking in oxygenated blood) or because the muscle has died and been replaced by scar. It shows the thickness or thinness of the ventricular wall and outlines ventricular *aneurysms*, or areas of blow-outs, similar to weak spots in the inner tube of a tire. It also details the condition of the valves guarding the entrance and exit of this heart chamber.

The film is processed and projected on a screen where viewers may study the condition of the interior of each coronary pipeline as well as the activity of the heart itself.

Cine coronary arteriography does not show all the disease that may be present and lesions that do not completely obstruct an artery may be missed. But narrow or completely obstructed arteries can usually be distinguished from normal pipelines. Arteriography determines with reasonable accuracy the location of the disease. It also indicates, among other things, which coronary artery is sufficiently free to allow passage of the blood to the heart, (Fig. 11), also the condition of the walls of the ventricles.

The final diagnosis for all disease rests with the pathological laboratory and the decision of the pathologist. A shadow shown by X ray on the upper part of the lung cannot be termed a cancer until that portion of the lung in which there was a shadow has been removed and sent to the pathologist for examination. The same is true of a lump in the breast which today can be shown most clearly by X ray or through a process called *thermography*. The films may indicate a cancer in the breast but the final diagnosis rests with the removal of the lump and its study by a pathologist.

The same point can be made in the area of heart disease. A true estimate of the extent and distribution of coronary artery disease is to be found not in the reports of cine arteriographers but in the studies of pathologists in autopsy rooms. Thus the surgeon operating to revascularize a heart often discovers at surgery more disease in heart muscle and in coronary arteries than was shown by electrocardiograms or by cine coronary arteriography.

It is a fact that the full ravages of coronary disease often come to light only in autopsy. It is also a fact that constantly-improving diagnostic procedures are making it possible to detect disease before it is too late. A veritable army of North Americans are alive today because their doctors were able to diagnose their illness.

CHAPTER 4

Stress — The Rat Race and Your Heart

Stress is insidious. It affects everyone at one time or another, and unfortunately seems to stalk certain individuals through most of their lives. It can inflict on its victims the pain of stomach ulcers, bowel irritations, and heart attacks. In some instances, it can trigger death.

A certain amount of stress may be good for you, as some have suggested, but its inherent dangers for the potential heart disease victim are many and they have been well documented.

As far back as the late nineteenth century, the famous Sir William Osler, of McGill University and John Hopkins University, drew attention to the importance of stress as a causative factor in the development of coronary artery atherosclerosis. And research since has confirmed the observation.

Stress can elevate blood pressure in certain people and the results of this are well defined:

> Worry a lot and your blood pressure may rise.
> Work under constant tension and your blood pressure could become dangerously high.

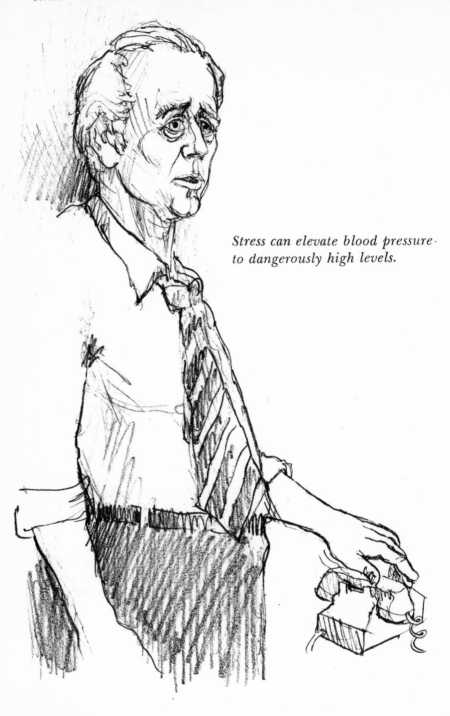

Stress can elevate blood pressure to dangerously high levels.

Stress is one of the risk factors in coronary heart disease, but to understand the full extent to which it can affect the heart, we must recognize that it is frequently associated to a greater or lesser degree with one or more of the other major risk elements.

We are all familiar with the plaintive cry of the bereaved widow, "His job finally killed him." Stress alone may not have brought on death but it might well have been the proverbial straw that broke the camel's back. Let us assume, for example, that the coronary arteries of the individual in question have been narrowed by fatty deposits. Add stress to this condition and the danger of a heart attack increases.

The explanation is that stress increases the heart rate (frequency of heart beat). The heart muscle, beating faster, needs more oxygenated blood which it cannot get because the coronary arteries are narrowed. With time, the heart muscle supplied by the narrowed arteries may become paralyzed and stop contracting. The patient has angina over the next few hours (or days) and part of the heart muscle may then die and the person has a heart attack.

In case of diabetes mellitus, a metabolic disease in which sugars and fats circulating in the blood stream are not properly utilized, stress is especially dangerous. The patient lives, so to speak, in double jeopardy.

By its very nature, diabetes mellitus upsets the metabolism, the process involved in changing food and other substances taken into the body into tissue, or converting them into energy. Fatty substances in the blood such as cholesterol and triglycerides are improperly utilized, resulting in atherosclerosis.

Diabetes is, of course, a disease in its own right but there is more than just a casual relationship between it and heart disease. In fact, it is widely acknowledged that two out of three patients with diabetes eventually develop cardiovascular diseases.

It becomes clear then that a diabetic, with his proneness to coronary artery disease, must assiduously avoid any stress that may add even the slightest burden to his already overtaxed arterial system.

Stress works cunningly in conjunction with other hazards and this is where it becomes difficult to identify. When a person is under stress, he is frequently a victim of fatigue. Tiredness, of course, robs an individual of the desire for one of nature's great therapies— physical activity. Without sufficient exercise, one runs the risk of becoming overweight. And carrying extra weight around is one of the coronary risk factors.

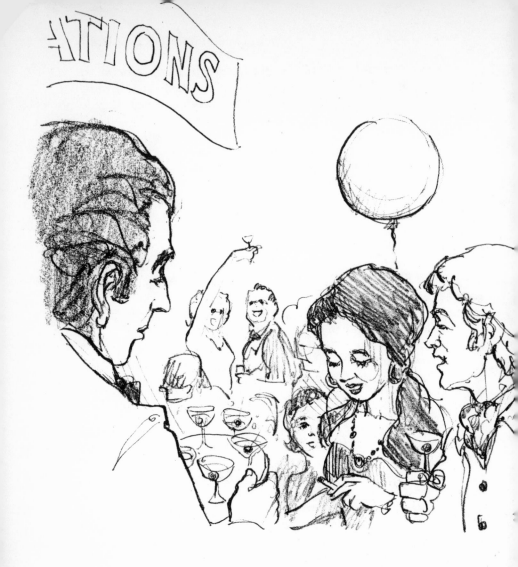

Cigarettes and Alcohol

Of all the risk factors for coronary artery heart disease, smoking may well be one of the worst, if not indeed *the* worst. It affects the nervous system, the lungs, and the heart. Its most serious effect, however, is on the circulation. Evidence indicates that people who smoke cigarettes develop a substance in their blood that increases the rate of clotting.

Smoking might bring on a heart condition but in the background there may also lurk the element of stress, so well camouflaged as to be hardly identifiable.

Thus, the stress-cigarette smoking combination is a vicious

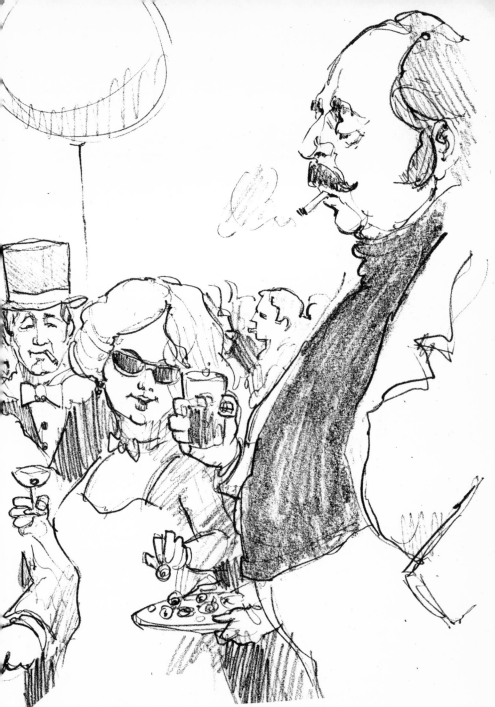

Smoking is probably the highest risk factor for coronary heart disease. Alcohol can be relaxing, but excessive use adds to stress of life.

circle, snaring the unwitting individual. The person under stress reaches for a cigarette in the belief that it offers relaxation. Instead, it irritates the nervous system. Newly agitated, he or she reaches for another cigarette, and another. Instead of finding relaxation, the person is actually building up more tension.

The tense individual, seeking relief from stress by smoking, is really further constricting arteries that may already be dangerously narrowed.

Smoking is one risk you can eliminate. I have heard all the arguments about how hard it is to quit but the fact is that it *can* be done.

Stop smoking.

I make the point categorically, without reservations. Stop— and you may add years to your life. Keep on lighting cigarettes and you may well be committing suicide. Remember, smoking will not alleviate stress. It will augment it.

What about alcohol, you ask? Should it be on the taboo list along with cigarettes?

My answer is that *some* people should abstain. Diabetics, for example, should not drink because alcohol raises the body's blood sugar levels and they already have a problem coping with elevated sugar concentrations. People subject to high blood pressure should also stay away from liquor. It sometimes has an adverse effect on hypertension.

If there are no special contraindications, however, my advice is simple: if you enjoy a drink, go ahead and have it. But don't drink to excess. Quite simply, if you can relax over a drink or two, liquor is probably good for you. I have even recommended it to some patients.

On the other hand, if you're the kind of person who drowns his problems in liquor every night, you may be in trouble. Apart from the damage you may do to your liver and kidneys, you will also be adding stress to your life. Doing a day's work after a night's drinking is a sure way of increasing tension.

"I knew a man who drank 40 ounces of whiskey every single day of his adult life and he never knew what it was like to be sick," a man once told me defiantly. Well, that could be true. In fact, I, too, once knew such a man. He'd have 16 ounces under his belt before lunch and put another 16 there before dinner. Then, as the comic said, he'd get down to some serious drinking all with no admitted ill effects. But I want to stress that these cases are exceptions.

Is there, then, such a thing as a *safe* amount?

Doctors do not usually recommend dosages of liquor, but if you're not diabetic, or suffering from high blood pressure, 4 ounces a day should be harmless. Since it takes one hour for the body to metabolize one ounce of liquor, there is no danger of overtaxing the system's chemical processes.

Psychological Aspects of Stress

So much for the medical aspects of stress but now, what about the psychological aspects?

For the heart doctor, the latter, with its myriad complications is a vital area of study.

Stress is a part of modern living, we're told. There is no way of avoiding it. It is something to be accepted as inevitable, a condition with which one must cope.

"But how do I cope with stress?" a patient wants to know.

"You don't let things get you down," I advise.

The words are scarcely out of my mouth, of course, when I realized the emptiness of my counsel. If my patient were able to ignore his problems, he wouldn't be in his present state.

Yet there is a lot you can do for yourself. With some effort, you can *train* yourself to ride out the stresses of life. For instance:

> Make up your mind not to let every annoying telephone call upset you.
>
> Resolve not to construe every remark your employer makes as a personal affront. (There's a good chance he meant nothing by the remark.)
>
> Don't get upset by every little argument that crops up in your household.

It's simple advice really and if you heed it, you'll be on the road to coping with the trials and tribulations of life.

Kevin B., one of my patients, is a good example. Ambitious and aggressive, he worked day and night to build up his business, and rarely found a moment for relaxation. Vacations were out of the question. There was always something to be done. He carried on like this until the day he felt great pain. (Kevin was the patient who described the pain by saying it felt as if an elephant was sitting on his chest.) His left arm went numb, but he managed to ease himself into a chair, and for a long time, sitting there clutching his chest and arm, he thought he was going to die.

I operated on Kevin and he came through well but he did a lot of thinking after that. In fact, he rethought his whole existence. He now realized how precious his life really was, and set about re-establishing his priorities. You should hear him now:

"I used to get so tense. Sometimes I thought I'd explode. There were always problems, and I always met them head on. Crash! I can see now that I went about almost everything in the wrong way."

"You must still have to contend with many tensions in your business, don't you?" I ask.

"Of course," he says. "You can't run a business without it. But I've changed my attitudes. I don't worry about things the way I used to."

He makes it all sound so simple:

"I've made up my mind I'm not going to let things get me down. I'm not going to get up-tight every time the work starts piling up. I'm not going to fret because I'm not punctual for an appointment. If I can't get there at two o'clock, I'll phone and say I'll be there at three. When I feel the tension mounting now, I simply shrug and say, 'The hell with it.'"

I was pleased to hear him say this because he was echoing my own antidote. *The hell with it.* Well, of course. That's the answer. It's that simple. If a person is able to say this when things go wrong, he can probably save himself a whole lot of grief.

Stress is one of the great intangibles of medical science. It takes so many different forms and strikes in so many different ways. You never can be sure just what effect it will have on any one particular individual.

There are two kinds of stress, physical and mental, and the danger is that a person may fall victim to either with little or no warning.

A doctor usually has little trouble coming to grips with a case of physical stress. For example, when a sedentary office worker tells you that his attack occurred while he was shoveling the driveway, you can pretty safely trace the stress factor back to the unaccustomed work he was doing. Again, if a man tells you the pain came while playing tennis on a very hot day, it's not too difficult to identify the cause.

Mental stress is a different proposition. Particularly with patients with angina or previous heart attacks, you are faced with a less clearly defined situation. A wife tells you that she did every-

Physical stress caused by playing tennis on a very hot day, for example, is not difficult to identify. Mental stress is a different proposition.

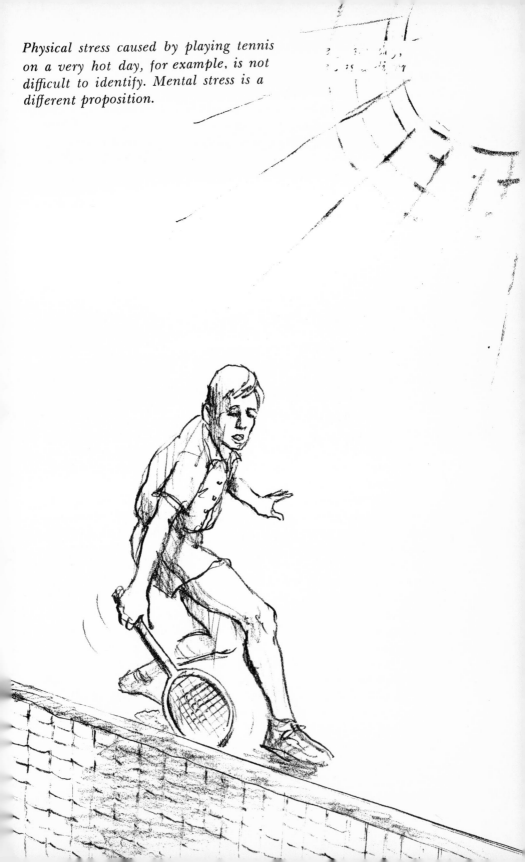

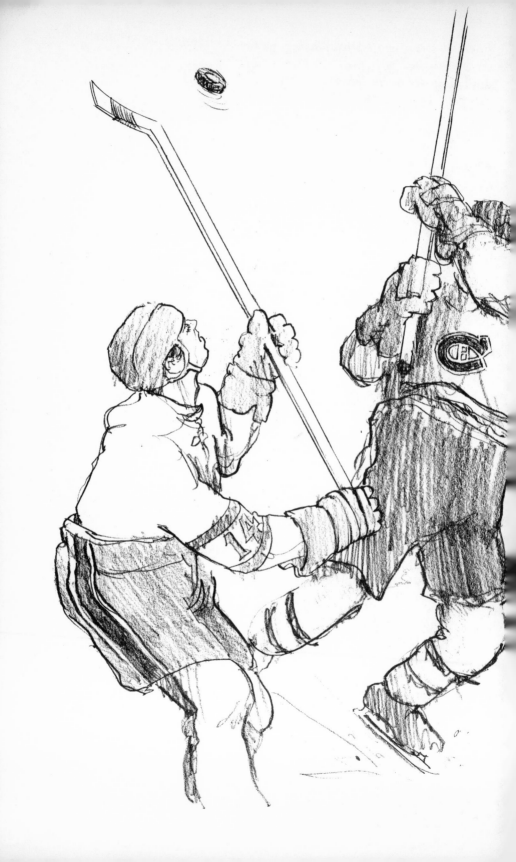

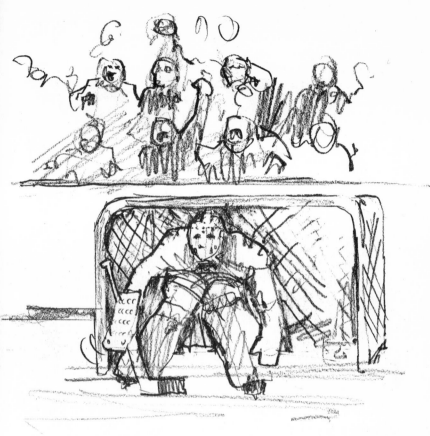

For some heart disease patients, the stress and excitement of watching a highly competitive sport can cause a heart attack.

thing, absolutely everything, to protect her husband against another heart attack. She wouldn't let him shovel, she says. She wouldn't let him lift the groceries out of the trunk of the car. She wouldn't let him walk in very cold weather. Then one day, without warning, he slumps over in great pain—right in front of the television set.

You probe further and find the man was watching a hockey game. Well, hockey is a lot of fun—but some people take their fun pretty seriously. This man did and on the evening in question, he got particularly excited and suffered a heart attack.

Why? Well, as I say, we're dealing with intangibles but this man had had a previous attack, his coronary arteries had become

71

narrowed and the tension of the game simply pushed him beyond his stress-tolerance level. The excitement of the game had sent his blood pressure up, thus triggering the attack.

The patient's wife had difficulty understanding this. If her husband had been playing the game, it might have made sense. The exertion could well have been too much for him. But he was *watching* the game, not *playing* it.

What I said next confused her even more. I would expect, I said, more casualties among the spectators at a sports event than among the players.

Certainly the players are in a state of acute stress. The condition increases their blood pressures and heart rates and elevates their blood sugars. These sugars, however, are burned up in sports combat. The man sitting at home in front of the television screen, on the other hand, may also find himself in a situation of stress with elevated blood sugar levels—and have no opportunity of bringing them down with physical activity, thus triggering a heart attack.

At the risk of unnecessarily alarming the Saturday afternoon audience of males watching sports in their living rooms, I must note that watching television can elevate blood sugars in some people. A tense cops-and-robbers film can raise the blood sugars as easily as a crucial game of football or baseball.

We humans are a varied lot. Some of us are capable of enduring a great deal of stress in our lives, and others can take very little.

How would you, for instance, react in the following situation?

The telephone rings. You pick it up and a serious voice tells you that your son has been injured in an automobile accident. It looks bad, the voice says, and perhaps you should hurry to the hospital.

If your body responses could be monitored at just this point, certain definite rhythmic changes would be recorded. Your blood pressure and heart rate, for example, likely would be up. So would your blood sugars.

Would you be able to cope with the shock?

If you were in reasonably good physical shape, chances are you would. Your pumping heart muscle, however, would be carrying an extra load and would require a compensating supply of blood. If your coronary arteries had become narrowed, it might not be possible for sufficient blood to get through. When the heart muscle doesn't get an adequate supply of blood, part of it dies. This is when you have a heart attack.

We are faced with many questions in dealing with stress. Why is it that one person can cope with it, and another can't? Why is it

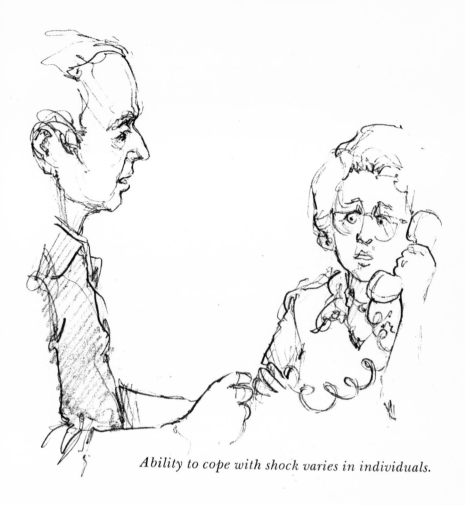

Ability to cope with shock varies in individuals.

that one man does his best work when he is under the gun, while another simply becomes ineffective, and even ill, under pressure?

We don't have all the answers. We do know, however, that stress has no respect for social or economic groups. We know about busy executives and their susceptibility to heart attacks. Every time you pick up a newspaper, you see the name of some prominent person, a company president perhaps, who died suddenly, or suffered a serious attack.

Teachers and professors face stress too, as do many students, particularly during examinations. Doctors and surgeons working around the clock, lawyers meeting the challenge of the courtroom— they too, are under stress much of their lives.

We tend to think of victims of stress-provoked heart attacks as coming strictly from the so-called white-collar classes but this is not so. For instance, truck drivers often work under conditions of great tension and have a high incidence of heart attacks. Today, even the street cleaner falls prey to stress. In the days of the horse and carriage, his life was leisurely, less perilous. Under modern conditions, working in the midst of high-speed traffic, he must be constantly alert to avoid serious injury or death.

In fact, the automobile itself has contributed to the high incidence of stress in everyday life. The salesman, forced to travel by car from city to city, coping with adverse weather and road conditions, is under a great deal of stress. So is the commuter, who has to fight city traffic morning and night. He has an added strike against him: he spends so much time in his car, he is in generally poor physical condition from lack of exercise.

Today's law-enforcement officer is, of course, an obvious example of a man under stress. Not only does he risk his life at the hands of the criminal element but he is also under fire from society and the courts. It is no wonder that there is such a high incidence of heart disease among police officers.

Nor is the housewife immune to the tensions of modern living. The care of young children, the rigors of coping with everyday problems around the home, the rising cost of living—all of these cause stress. Added to this, the housewife worries about her husband, and what his job is doing to *his* health.

Stress is not related solely to one's employment or occupation. For many, there is the stress of financial worry—how to meet the mortgage payment, how to finance the children's education. Concern over an illness in the family or a child's behavior can also increase the dangers already entailed by the stress of one's occupation.

Many refuse to admit it but often there is considerably more stress on the home front than in the office or factory. Many a husband or wife has found blessed relief from tension simply by getting out of the house! A short walk, or, better still, if one's up to it, a long walk, will do wonders when it comes to lowering blood sugar levels and restoring calm.

Effects of Stress on the Heart

Research into the relationship between stress and the heart has produced some interesting results at Memorial Hospital Medical Center in Long Beach, California.

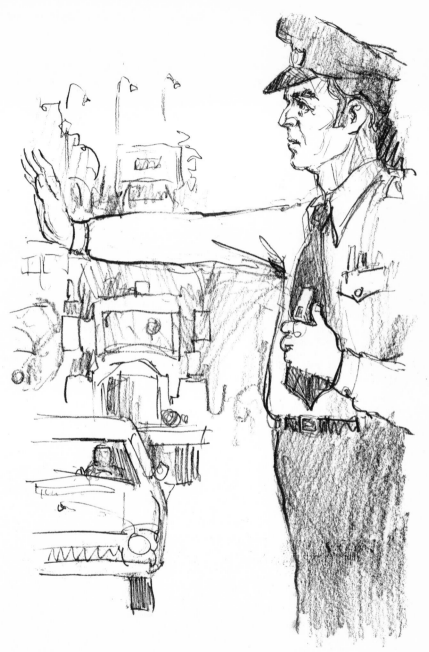

Stress is believed to have led to the high incidence
of heart disease among police officers.

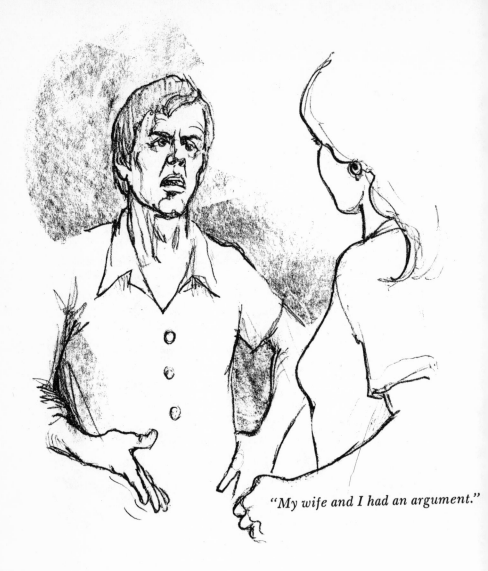

"*My wife and I had an argument.*"

Doctors there have been experimenting with what they call the *10-hour dynamic electrocardiograph.* Each patient wears a box about the size of a small portable radio, attached to ECG electrodes taped to the chest. He is instructed to engage in his normal activity. The next day, a doctor examines the results. In ten minutes, he reviews the entire 10-hour ECG tape and is able to pinpoint abnormalities in heart activity and the time they occurred.

Cardiologist William Allen explains that the usual ECG is recorded in three minutes, while the patient is resting, and away from the stresses of job and home but the *dynamic* ECG records 600 minutes of actual daily living. Extra beats and abnormal rhythms are quickly spotted. Once he pinpoints a problem, the physician calls for a print-out of the trouble area on the tape. (This is done quickly on a special machine.)

"Where were you and what were you doing at 5:30 yesterday afternoon?" Dr. Allen asks his patient, after spotting an abnormality on the tape which appears to indicate some disturbance at that time.

"I was driving home," the patient recalls. "It was rush hour. The traffic was terrible." He pauses, remembering the incident. "Somebody cut me off and I got mad."

Dr. Allen says that the 10-hour ECG is especially valuable in letting a physician know if a heart patient is ready to drive his car after a heart attack or after surgery. The ECG may show an abnormal rhythm or a change indicating that the heart is not getting enough blood. But if the patient can drive down the street without revealing any abnormalities, this is solid evidence that it's all right for him to stay behind the wheel.

The ECG is an excellent instrument for determining whether or not a person is capable of facing physical and emotional stresses. Taping a housewife in her own home, for instance, provides doctors with information that tests done in a hospital would not provide. It also proves valuable in the case of the person who suffers fainting spells which may or may not be caused by a heart ailment. If it *is* the heart, the ECG will enable the physician to determine this by revealing what abnormal rhythms occurred at the time of each episode.

The tests sometimes provide surprises. In one case a doctor, worried about a patient returning to an extremely stress-provoking occupation, called for an ECG that would record his heart activity during the first day back on the job. The following day, the doctor, reviewing the tape, was surprised and puzzled to find that the man had made it through a particularly hectic day with no problems. But at 6 P.M. an abnormal rhythm was recorded.

"Was it the result of an accumulation of pressures?" the doctor wondered aloud. "What happened at six o'clock last night?"

The patient grinned. "My wife and I had an argument," he reported.

CHAPTER 5

Sex and Your Heart

Sexual intercourse is a healthy and necessary part of living—and this is as true of the middle-aged individual who has had coronary artery heart disease as it is of the healthy, younger person.

I shall go a step further: the happiness and well-being of a person in the postcoronary period sometimes *depends* on his ability to handle his sexuality.

I can understand the worries and fears of the heart disease victim. Naturally, he is concerned about his ability to return to a normal way of life. But it is wrong for people to resign themselves to meager, dull lives as cardiac cripples. I have seen altogether too many of these cripples, people afraid to stray from their easy chairs, frightened to go out of the house because of what *might* happen.

A heart attack does not have to mean an end to life; neither should it necessarily signal an end to a man's sexual role. This is not to say there are no pitfalls. There are certain risks and you should be aware of them.

For example, sexual intercourse can bring on anginal pain in some individuals. (A Cleveland study suggests one in five postcoronary subjects experiences pain in love-making.) In extreme cases, sex can even trigger death.

When I refer to cardiac cripples, I have in mind that life is full of calculated risks. The point is that it is essential for a person's

*A heart attack need not signal
the end to a man or woman's
sexual role.*

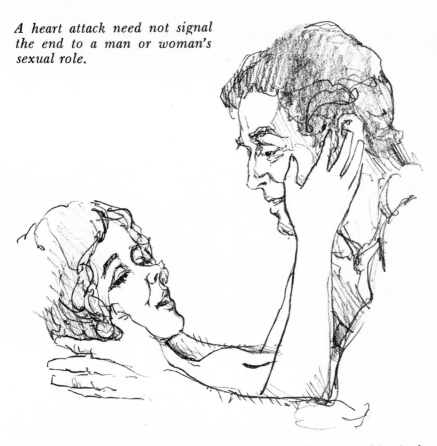

spiritual well-being to live as full and normal a life as possible. And just as it is necessary for a heart victim to return to some useful form of employment, so it is also necessary for him to fulfill his role as husband and lover.

What then are the real facts? Is sex dangerous for men in the coronary age group, and is it particularly hazardous for those who have actually had heart attacks?

Generalizations are meaningless, so I'll stay away from them. I shall resort rather to common sense as it applies to the individual. Let me put it this way: treat sex in the same way you would any other physical activity.

If you're soft, flabby, and 60, it could be dangerous for you to play a fast game of tennis singles. It would be equally dangerous at

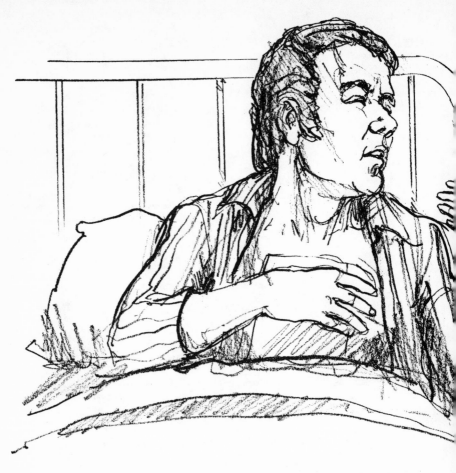

John's attractive girl friend had visited him.

that age and in that condition for you to try to satisfy the sexual appetite of a 21-year-old woman.

Research in the area of sexual excitement as it affects the cardiac case is limited but I have had a number of examples in my own practice.

I am reminded of a young patient named John who came to me a couple of years ago with a leaking heart valve. He was in his late twenties and one of the youngest people on whom I ever operated.

The operation was a success and the signs were all good. John appeared on the way to recovery. Then, 48 hours after the operation, there was an emergency. His pulse became very rapid and he

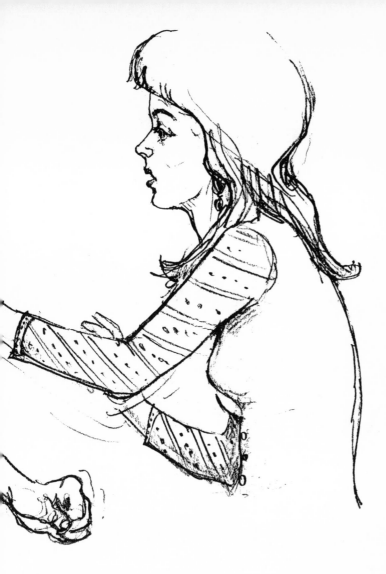

was short of breath. He finally went into a state of complete collapse. Our hospital people fortunately were able to bring him back and John made a full recovery.

I was puzzled. I couldn't understand why there had been complications. I learned the reason from a nurse. John's highly-attractive girl friend had visited him. She sat down on the bed and he put his arms around her and kissed her. That brought on the emergency.

North American males are not noted as great lovers. Nonathletic in a great many cases, beset by domestic and business problems, they tend to slip into a condition of sexual apathy in their middle years.

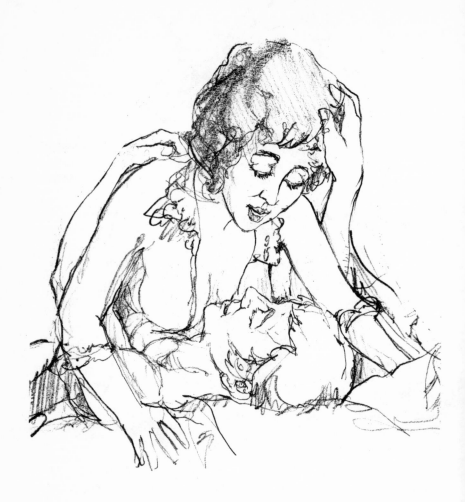

Yet the subject of sex comes up with amazing regularity in most of my interviews—"Will I be able to make love to my wife again?" a patient wants to know after his operation. His worried wife, on the other hand, poses another question: "Would it be better if we didn't make love?"

I am quite candid with my patients. I tell them that in all probability they will be able to resume their sexual activities—and enjoy them quite as much as they did before their operations.

It may take time, of course. You can't hurry things after an operation. A patient improves at his own pace and in his own time. It could be several weeks, or for that matter several months. (One U.S. study shows that the average period of abstinence is about 14 weeks, although relations may be resumed sooner by subjects who had a strong sex drive prior to the coronary onset.)

Actually, the average middle-aged North American male uses about the same amount of oxygen during intercourse as he does going for a short, brisk walk, climbing a flight of stairs, or performing simple jobs at his place of employment.

You can resume your sex life when you find that you are capable of performing ordinary home tasks and are able to engage in some physical activity. If you can do exercise that uses 6–8 calories per minute, as in vigorous walking for one hour, without abnormal pulse rate or blood pressure levels, you can safely perform the sex act.

If your sex drive appears to be waning, then there may be other reasons. Many patients with heart conditions also have diabetes mellitus with impotence. You might fall into this category. Again, you may be taking antihypertensive medication which can interfere with sexual performance. The fear of impotence can be a very grave factor and actually curtail a person's sex life seriously.

You may become very worried about your sexual ability, and in later phases of recovery minor tranquilizers may help relieve your anxiety.

The short-acting effect of alcohol may also be of value to the man who is anxious about his performance. But note that barbiturates may depress sex. Thus, judicious use of alcohol or tranquilizers may produce enough relaxation to ensure the success of a patient's first postcoronary attempt at sex and thus avoid a possible chronic sex problem in the future.

If the heart is lacking a sufficient supply of blood, sex may bring on anginal pain. This is less likely to occur if one has sex on an empty stomach. Sex before dinner? Yes, it's much safer that way.

Do *not* engage in sexual activity right after a meal. It is unwise to do brisk exercise, even vigorous walking, for an hour and a half after eating, and usually I advise my patients to allow a full two hours.

Don't push yourself if you're tired. Wait. Fatigue is bad for an ailing heart. Some people like sex relations in the morning when the body is rested. This, and weekends, are better for intercourse than late evenings if you have a coronary problem.

83

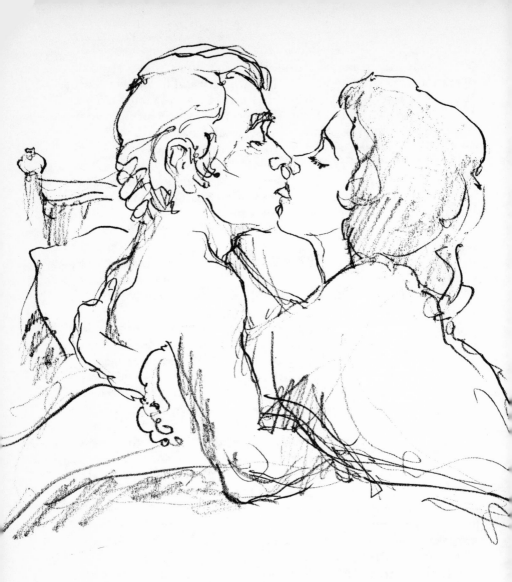

The man with the heart condition who finds the sex act arduous should perhaps try different positions. There are many positions in which the act can be performed and variations tend to give new zest and interest to intercourse.

Some of my patients have found the traditional male dominant position too strenuous to assume after a coronary. In these cases I recommend that the woman assumes the dominant position. Female dominant? Woman on top? Why not? It's an interesting variation.

Some couples have discovered they enjoy intercourse lying on their sides. However, coronary patients must be careful about lying on their left side (which puts pressure on the heart). They may lie on their right side with ease.

For some cardiac patients, sexual activity poses a serious problem. For others, it doesn't. Dr. Cornelius B. Bakker, of the University of Washington in Seattle, says that the trauma of heart disease lies in its capacity to undermine the patient's confidence in his strength and vigor. This sense of inadequacy enhances the fear of sexual intercourse, leading to impotence.

Dr. Bakker makes another point and that is that it's extremely important for the physician to include the wife in any counseling session with a heart patient. It is not sufficient just to tell the patient that he can have sexual relations. It is important that the wife realizes that it is perfectly safe to do so.

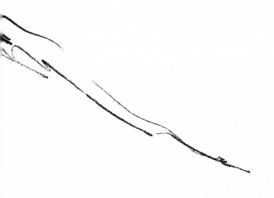

CHAPTER 6

Food and Your Heart

The great search for good health, particularly in North America and Western Europe, has produced some highly intriguing nutritional habits in the last few years—and a profusion of confusion about what to eat and what *not* to eat.

High fat diet or low fat diet? Which should it be? Both have been recommended at one time or another. Calories? We have been told to count them and *not* to count them. We have been urged to try the grapefruit diet, the banana diet, the no-food diet of water and vitamins. We have even catered to the martini crowd with a drinking man's diet.

The plans all aim at weight reduction and for the great number of overweight people in our society, the objective is valid even if the means are open to argument.

Who are the overweight people of our affluent society? Well, certainly not only the affluent. Being fat doesn't necessarily mean you are well nourished. There is much overweight with malnutrition found among low-income North Americans, and particularly among those without work. Not only do these people not eat the proper foods but too many of them spend their days in a sedentary position in front of the television set.

And herein lies the key to understanding the relationship between diet and good health.

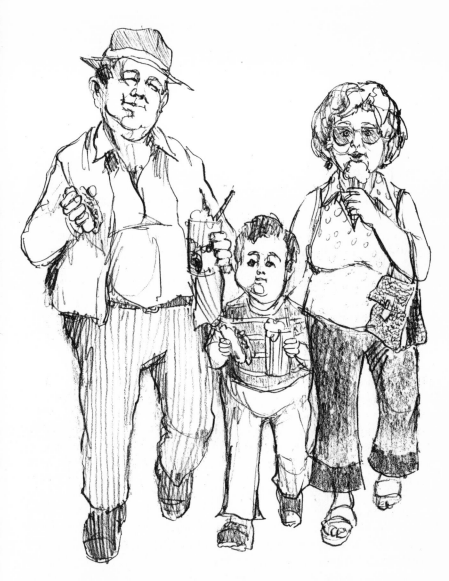

Being fat doesn't necessarily mean you are well nourished.

While the objective of weight reduction is important, you must be sure that the diet you choose does not lead to malnutrition. You must also be sure that it doesn't raise the cholesterol in your system to dangerous levels.

Working out a diet that leaves you well-fed while allowing you to keep your weight in control may be one of the most important things you do for your heart.

You must not allow yourself to become fat because the dangers to your heart are just too great. The facts speak for themselves: Obesity is associated with high blood pressure and diabetes, both of which are risk factors in coronary artery disease. In addition, population studies have shown that serum cholesterol values tend to mirror weight gain. High serum cholesterol combined with high blood pressure increases the risk of coronary artery disease five-fold.

There is a direct relationship between obesity and atherosclerosis. If you take on excess body fat, you will put a strain on your cardiovascular system. You will tire more easily, thus reducing your capacity for work and physical activity. The problem will be compounded because your inability to exercise will only produce still more body weight.

The true causes of obesity, if glandular factors are excluded, are still a matter of controversy. Many modern medical authorities agree that overfeeding a baby in the first six months of life leads to an excess of fat cells in the body. The theory is that when an over-fed child becomes an adult, he must struggle constantly to prevent the fat cells from filling up.

Other researchers cite heredity in explanation. If the parents are fat, they maintain, so usually are the children. While genetic incidence of obesity does occur, I believe it is frequently true that obese youngsters are victims of insufficient exercise and poor eating habits, both of which are acquired through parental example.

There is a great deal that can be done to prevent coronary artery disease and general atherosclerosis, but we must examine the whole picture and not just part of it.

As you read on, you will begin to understand that diet alone simply is not enough. It must be combined with an effective exercise program and even that is not enough. The type of diet chosen must be a cholesterol-conscious diet, and should be composed of about 25 percent of unsaturated fatty acids. The chart that I have prepared (which appears at the end of this book) could very well be the most important guide to eating you could ever follow.

Before we discuss specific diets, let me first emphasize that no diet program, no matter how scientific, can stand alone. Exercise

Children are frequently victims of insufficient exercise and poor eating habits.

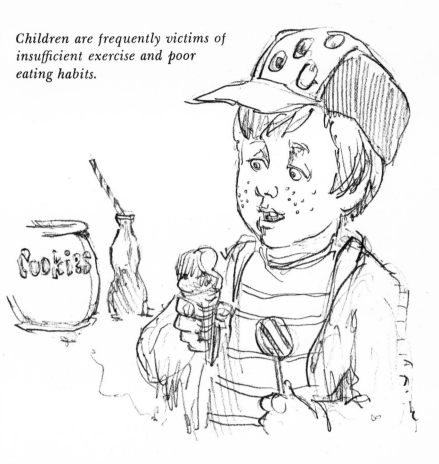

must be a part of it. Exercise increases a person's metabolic rate, and thus calories are burned up. Furthermore, the increased metabolic rate is sustained over a 24-hour period, so that calories are burned up, not only during active exercise but over the full day. The exercise chapter of this book details the kind of exercise you should become involved in.

Now back to diets. Many people are confused about calories. The simple fact, however, is that people need a certain number of calories to meet the requirements of their daily activities.

Caloric needs vary a good deal. Women need only four-fifths the number of calories that men require. The surrounding temperature also plays a role. When it's cold, there is a greater heat loss and a need for more calories. In warm weather, you need fewer calories.

Calorie charts are widely available. Use them. They can tell you how many calories you need to fulfill your energy requirements and how to maintain your ideal weight on good *nutritional* food.

What is an ideal weight? I ask my patients how much they weighed at age 25, that is, when they were in good condition, with little or no fat. I tell them then that they should be within five to ten pounds of that weight.

So far so good. Getting the right number of calories through a selection of good, wholesome food is important. But that is only part of the story. You must also be aware of the biggest dietary killer of all—cholesterol. It is what we in modern medicine have come to

Exercise will help reduce blood cholesterol.

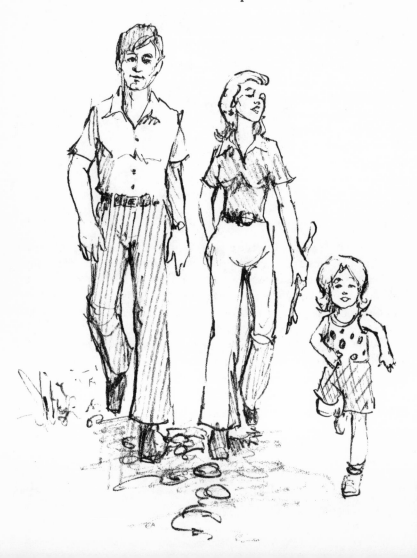

regard as one of the major factors in the development of coronary artery disease.

What exactly *is* cholesterol and how can we avoid it in food?

Certain facts have been well documented. We know that it is one of the complex cyclical alcohols known as sterols. We know that it is synthesized by the body and functions in normal metabolic processes. We know that it is present in all of the cells of the body and particularly in the liver, kidneys, brain, and pancreas. We believe that it is manufactured by the liver, adrenal cortex, skin, intestines, testis, and aorta.

Only foods of animal origin contain significant amounts of cholesterol, but trace amounts have been reported in plant tissue. It is found in the lipid fraction of animal tissues and may occur bound with protein as a lipoprotein. (A lipid is any one of a group of organic substances which are insoluble in water but soluble in alcohol, ether, chloroform, and other fat solvents that have a *greasy* feel. It embraces fatty acids and soaps, neutral fats, waxes, steroids, and phosphatides.)

Cholesterol is present in all animal cells and is necessary in the human body for the production of certain enzymes and various endocrine secretions. However, if the food one eats contains an excess of cholesterol, the body may not be able to handle it and the result may be an elevated blood cholesterol level.

To know where you stand, it is important for you to have your blood cholesterol and other lipoproteins analyzed. You should do this once a year. This is particularly important if you have a family history of heart trouble or if you are overweight. If the analysis indicates elevated blood cholesterol levels, your physician should recommend further expert study.

We believe that exercise will reduce blood cholesterol. However, if your intake of cholesterol is very high, no amount of exercise or work is going to eliminate it.

The point is that unless you take remedial dietary steps, cholesterol will not be eliminated and will find its way into the walls of coronary arteries and the arteries going to the brain itself. Cholesterol crystals lying in tissues are irritating and are believed by most that if they remain in the arterial walls for long periods of time they set up inflammatory changes which lead to atherosclerosis.

It is interesting to note that the incidence of atherosclerosis, a disease characterized by high cholesterol deposits and leading in many cases to coronary heart disease, is very high in Finland. Now, the Finns are hard-working, they exercise a lot, and they are thin.

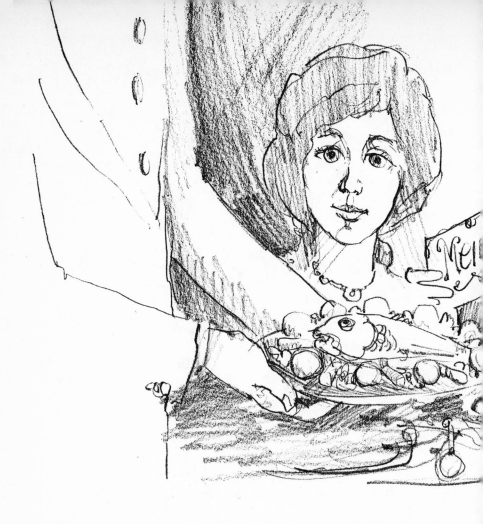

But they work in very cold weather, and in order to get energy, they rely a great deal on animal fats for the 5,000 calories they require every day in these cold temperatures. Their diet contains a high cholesterol content—and the fact that they are very active, and not overweight, does not spare them from atherosclerosis. It must be mentioned, of course, that the Finns have another coronary risk factor: they are heavy cigarette smokers.

The point is then that we must carefully watch what we eat. We must be sure, however, that our food is nutritious—and at the same time not high in cholesterol.

How much cholesterol may we safely take in our diets?

Dr. William B. Kannel, of the Framingham Heart Disease Epidemiology Study, sets these guidelines: for a healthy man or woman of ideal weight and getting adequate exercise: not more

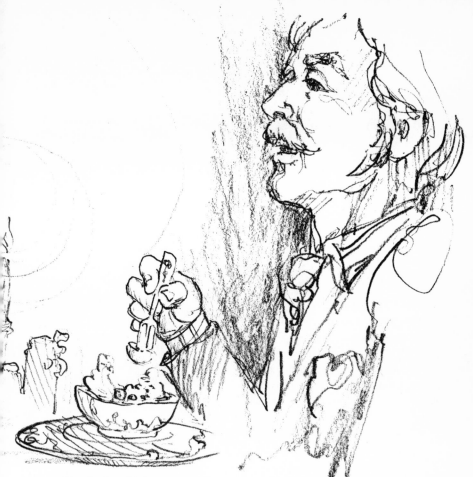

Food should be nutritious and low in cholesterol.

than 300 mg. a day; for the person with a family history of the disease 240 mg. a day.

It is worth noting, however, that in countries where blood cholesterol levels average 150 mg., there are practically no heart attacks. Perhaps then we should aim at cholesterol levels that are much lower than those accepted in North America.

On the basis of present evidence, I would recommend that we aim at blood cholesterol levels of below 180 mg.

Is is possible to enjoy a nutritious and varied diet on low cholesterol foods? It is indeed—and the chart is specifically designed to show you how.

The chart is divided into various subsections, such as dairy products, meats, vegetables, etc. The cholesterol content is given for each food product so you can easily note those with high concentrations. The caloric values are also noted. Hence, by selecting from the various groups of foods, it is possible to maintain a balanced nutritional diet and at the same time stay within your daily cholesterol guidelines.

For example, meats of all kinds contain cholesterol—but some cuts have more than others. Have a slice of roast beef, by all means. But stay clear of organ and glandular meats if you're thinking of cholesterol. Meats such as heart, kidney, liver, and sweetbreads have high concentrations, with the highest of all being found in brains.

Remember, cholesterol in food is not necessarily related to fat content, so don't assume that by removing fat, you are reducing cholesterol proportionately.

If you are a lover of seafood, you would do well, for example, to stay away from lobster Newburg. Remember, there are alternatives. Crab meat has less cholesterol than lobster. Shrimp has less than crab and scallops less than shrimp.

Here are a few other pointers:

Most fish (as distinguished from shell fish) are relatively low in cholesterol, while maintaining a high nutritional value. In most cases, you may enjoy generous portions without worry.

Fruit and vegetables also are low in cholesterol. At the same time they are high in numerous essential nutrients.

Egg yolks are high in cholesterol, so instead of having them every day, plan to have them only on special days, perhaps as a Sunday treat. In any event, limit your egg intake to four a week.

Generally, fats containing a high percentage of saturated fatty acids are solid or semi-solid. Those containing a high percentage of unsaturated fatty acids are liquids and largely found in vegetable and fish oils.

At present, saturated fats are believed by most authorities to raise blood cholesterol levels. Such fats contain a high percentage of saturated fatty acids. Fats and oils which contain a high percentage of monounsaturated fatty acids appear to have no effect on the blood cholesterol either way. Vegetable and fish oils contain a high percentage of polyunsaturated fatty acids except for coconut oil and palm kernel. Oils with a high content of polyunsaturated fatty acids are believed to play a part in lowering blood serum cholesterol levels. The body can use all types of fats but the total intake of fat should not make up more than 35 percent of the total daily calorie requirements. Of that amount it is recommended that 10 percent of the total calorie requirements should come from saturated fatty acids and 10 percent from polyunsaturated fatty acids with the balance of 15 percent from monounsaturated fatty acids.

It is thus desirable to eat fats and oils with a high percentage of polyunsaturated fatty acids and avoid those that contain a high percentage of saturated fatty acids such as butter. However, in replacing butter with margarine it is important that the margarine you buy contains a high percentage of polyunsaturated fatty acids. While there are excellent vegetable margarines on the market, in particular, corn oil and safflower oil, that fill this requirement, all do not, so be sure to check the package.

Become a skim milk family. Don't have whole milk in the house. Skim milk has all the nutrients that are present in whole milk, without the dangerous fat.

I know how difficult it is to stick with rules and I sympathize with people who really enjoy certain high cholesterol foods. I am one of them myself. But there is a healthy way out of this predicament. Limit yourself to a suitable cholesterol intake for periods of one week. In this way, you can enjoy certain high cholesterol foods —as long as you don't exceed your limit in any given week.

Study the chart. It's designed for you and your family. Make it your guide to good health. Watch out for low caloric foods which have been recommended in reducing diets but which have a high cholesterol content.

CHAPTER 7

Exercise and Your Heart

Physical culture has always been particularly susceptible to faddism and perhaps nowhere is this truer than in the United States and Canada. Millions of North Americans, warned repeatedly that they are a soft, flabby lot, today are getting on the fitness bandwagon, eager for a quick, simple formula for good health. They are flocking to gymnasiums to exercise muscles they have forgotten they had. They are rushing to handball and tennis courts for lunch-time workouts. Some are pushing themselves around parks in the great jogging spree.

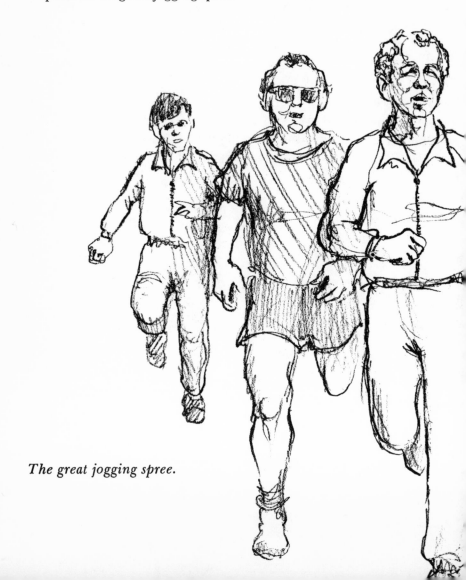

The great jogging spree.

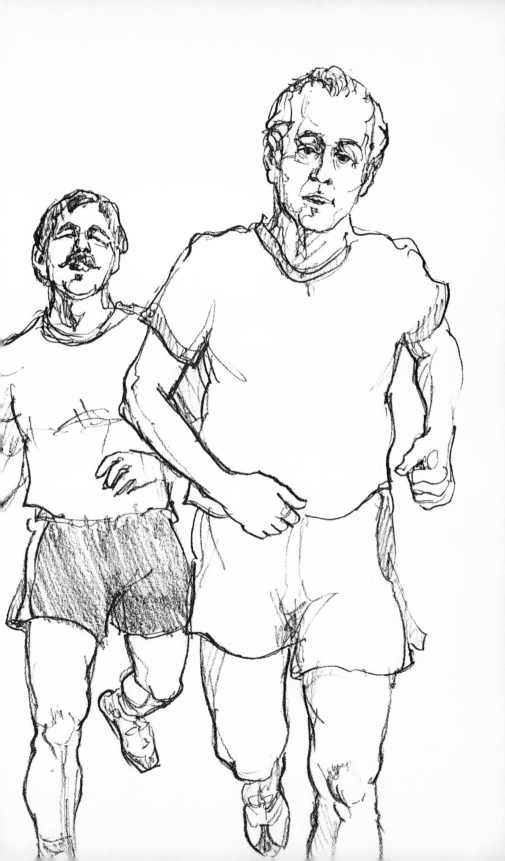

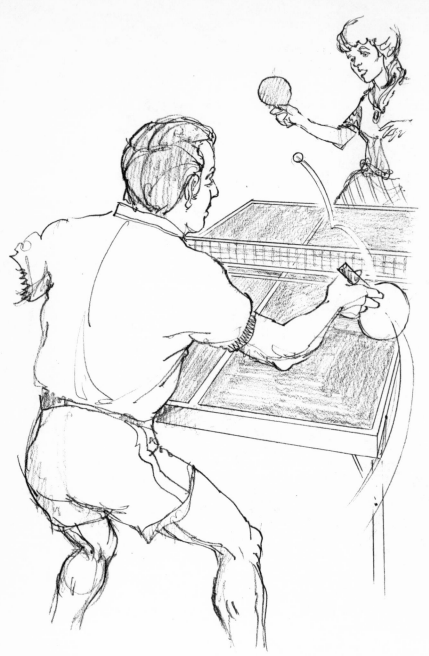

You don't necessarily have to take out a membership in a club to keep trim.

Oh what a worried lot they are—and is it any wonder? The good life of America has produced a high quota of what we might call *motionless* people, men and women who seldom, if ever, walk in the open air, who rarely climb stairs, swim, or play a game that requires physical movement. They have forgotten the simple joys of walking, of working up a sweat in the sandlot, of batting the bird across the badminton net in the backyard.

The critics are correct. The state of physical fitness is indeed woefully below par. The time has come to begin directing some physical activity back into our daily living to counteract the sloth and gluttony promoted by modern technology.

But remember, just as no program of diet is complete without exercise activity, no exercise program can be successful without attention to proper diet.

Gymnasiums are fine and I certainly have no quarrel with them. The good ones are generally well-equipped and offer safe, sophisticated programs. I have no quarrel either with the handball or tennis courts. What they serve up for lunch for tens of thousands of wise North Americans is a lot healthier than martinis, straight up or on the rocks.

Remember though that you don't necessarily have to take out a membership in a club to keep in trim. You don't have to pay money for a professional plan of action and you don't absolutely require special equipment. There are many other things you can do:

> Get out in the fresh air and walk briskly.
> As you walk, break into a little jog.
> Set up a badminton court in your backyard and use it.
> If there is water nearby, get a boat and try some good old-fashioned rowing.
> If you have a bicycle (and a safe place to ride it), do a few miles every evening.
> Work up a little sweat—but enjoy what you're doing.

Let us stop to examine the situation. Remember, not all exercise is good for all people. For instance snow shoveling can be dangerous. It puts a load on the heart and frequently precipitates a heart attack.

The human body has what are known as skeletal muscles, or organs of movement. They are responsible for all voluntary body movements, and compose 40 percent of the weight of the human body. Exercise designed to build up these muscles through daily isometric contractions, such as those in a strictly gymnasium-type

The right *kind of exercise is beneficial to the cardiovascular system.*

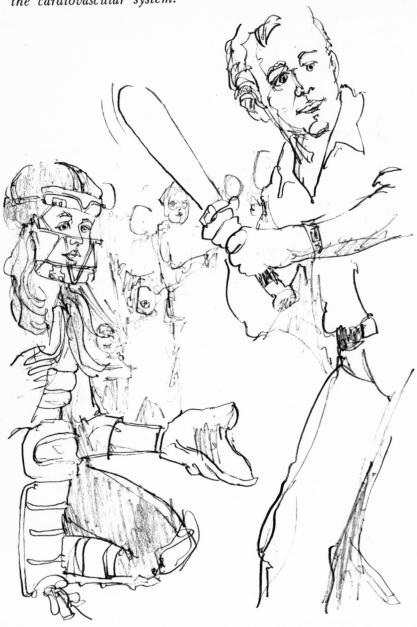

program may be good in terms of toning up muscles and keeping a flat stomach but they are said to do very little to condition the cardiovascular system. However, the famous Canadian 5BX plan is a valuable form of cardiovascular exercise because it combines muscle-toning isometric exercise with a regularly scheduled program of walking or jogging or running on the spot geared to the individual's age and physical capacity.

There is considerable evidence, however, to indicate that the right kind of exercise *is* beneficial to the cardiovascular system. It helps keep blood cholesterol levels down in the majority of people. This is of particular importance because as we have seen in the chapter on diet, an elevated blood cholesterol is one of the major contributing factors to coronary artery atherosclerosis.

Among the evidence are the results of an experiment carried out at a western university. Two groups of students, all of them freshmen, took part. They were all known to have the same coronary factors: family histories of elevated blood cholesterol and lipoprotein, diabetes, and hypertension.

Members of both groups had their blood cholesterol levels checked before the experiment. Then they were put on a high fat, high cholesterol, high calorie (over 4,000) diet. Group A was excused from all exercise. Group B students played hockey for one hour twice a week. At the end of three months, cholesterol levels were again checked. Some members of Group A showed elevated readings while the hockey-playing Group B members all showed a decrease. This was confirmed in a further study at Harvard University.

If two hours a week of exercise will keep the cholesterol level normal, or even just slightly lower, then one has to accept the value of physical activity among young people as possibly being one of the preventive factors in the development of atherosclerosis.

However, if we agree on the value of exercise for the young, should we conclude that physical activity is good also for older generations?

The answer is yes—with an added word of caution.

Man reaches full maturity at age 25. After this, his muscle power begins to diminish. By the time he is 40, he no longer is the man he was at 25, particularly with reference to his muscles and the condition of his heart and cardiovascular system.

Because of our *easy* North American way of life, the need to regain exercise habits such as walking and climbing stairs is real and urgent.

However, I tend to be extra cautious with older people since atherosclerosis is part of the aging process. For example, it may be dangerous for anyone who has always lived a sedentary existence to set himself a strenuous exercise program. Most of us are familiar with the business executive, in poor physical shape because of years of sedentary living, who puts himself through some grueling jogging paces and ends up dropping dead in the park.

In other words, while I highly recommend physical activity and have even made a table of suggestions for people without coronary artery disease, there are situations in which a doctor's counseling is required. Remember, coronary artery disease can reach an advanced stage without symptoms or physical findings to betray its presence. The doctor, by careful questioning can determine whether there is a family history suggesting the presence of coronary risk factors. He then should carry out an electrocardiogram at rest after exercise, and check for hypertension, an enlarged left ventricle, impaired glucose tolerance and hypercholesterolemia as well as hyperlipemia. People with such factors may still benefit from exercise but it should be less strenuous and more carefully supervised.

If the subject is a high-risk coronary candidate who has been sedentary for years, he should be encouraged to walk outside whenever possible at a speed that is comfortable to him, stopping when he develops anginal pain. At no time should he take nitroglycerine to walk through anginal pain, as has been recommended by many physicians across the country. He will be better to stop, take a nitroglycerine pill, and return home slowly. In this way, he can gradually increase his exercise. A word of counsel: such exercise should not be carried out on a cold day, nor should it be done sooner than an hour and a half after eating.

I am very much against testing patients in the high risk group, who have been sedentary for a long period, on a treadmill or bicycle ergometer as has been suggested, with enough exercise to bring the heart rate up to 150 per minute. There have been far too many accidents with this type of testing. It is hardly realistic to test the patient to a point where he has a cardiac arrest, even though trained personnel are present to resuscitate him.

The principle of walking slowly and increasing to a faster pace, on the other hand, allows the patient time to condition himself. The plan should be carried out with a dietary program aimed at weight reduction.

It might be appropriate here to add a note about the hazards of *severe* exercise. The hazards exist not only for high risk coronary subjects but for everyone, including young adults. Severe exercise includes a number of activities. For many, for instance, it might involve tennis, squash, or handball singles, games which might be played more safely in doubles. Certainly as a person grows older, he should be content to play doubles.

Severe exercise increases blood pressure, which is a danger in itself, but it also decreases blood flow to kidneys and stomach.

The blood storing function of the veins is well known. During exercise the veins contract. The blood depots thus become reduced and the effective amount of circulating blood is increased. Under basal, or resting, conditions, the cardiac output is most stable in the lying position and is about 4 or 5 liters or quarts, per minute.

In the transition from rest to exercise, the cardiovascular function undergoes remarkable changes. During the initial stage of rhythmic muscular work, the cardiac output increases, first rapidly and then more gradually, from the resting state and up to a *niveau,* or *steady* state, the level of which is set by the intensity of work. The niveau is reached at about the same time as the oxygen uptake levels off at *its* steady state.

Thus, there are two components in the kinetic adjustment of cardiac output to rhythmic muscular exercise, a fast one caused by a centrally induced nervous drive, and a slower secondary phase which may be a result of some unknown reflex mechanisms. The final level of cardiac output is closely related to the intensity of work.

In light and moderate work, the duration of the adaption phase lasts for one or two minutes. It is related to the intensity of work and becomes longer in heavy exercise. Fit subjects adapt more quickly to exercise than do unfit subjects.

The cardiac output is determined by the stroke volume and the frequency of heart beat (heart rate). Let me explain. The cardiac output represents the total output of the heart per minute. Thus, if the stroke volume is 70 milliliters per minute and the rate per minute is 70, then the cardiac output is 4.9 liters per minute. If the stroke volume increases, as it does with exercise, and the rate increases, there is a resulting marked increase in cardiac output.

At rest and in the supine position, the stroke volume of an adult nonathletic man is 70–90 ml., depending on the body size. (In women, it is usually 25 percent less.) As a result of the greater venous return which occurs in transition from rest to exercise in the upright position, the stroke volume increases rapidly, reaching a level which is maintained during exercise of 5–10 minutes. During strenuous rhythmic skeletal contractions, the blood flow increases between 15 and 20 times above the resting value.

In a normal resting man with a cardiac output of 5 liters per minute, the visceral organs (liver, kidneys, spleen, and gastrointestinal tract) receive about 2.5 liters per minute, or 50 percent of the cardiac output. During exercise, the kidneys may lose between 50 and 80 percent of this, the decrease being roughly related to the intensity of work.

The more severe the exercise the greater the percentage of cardiac output directed to the skeletal muscles at the expense of the visceral organs.

Strenuous exercise appears to affect the kidneys because of the markedly diminished blood flow. Early in the century, Dr. W. Collier, observing the condition of urine among college crew members in England, reported that practically every oarsman displayed albuminuria, or protein in the urine, at one time or another. The more severe the exercise, the more marked the evidence of disturbance of the renal function.

As for the stomach, strenuous exercise inhibits both the motor and secretory functions of this organ and the rate at which it empties its contents into the duodenum. The amount of exercise required to inhibit gastric function varies with the physical fitness of the individual. However, medical researchers J. M. H. Campbell, G. O. Mitchell, and A. T. W. Powell concluded as early as

Severe exercise should be avoided by those not in top physical condition.

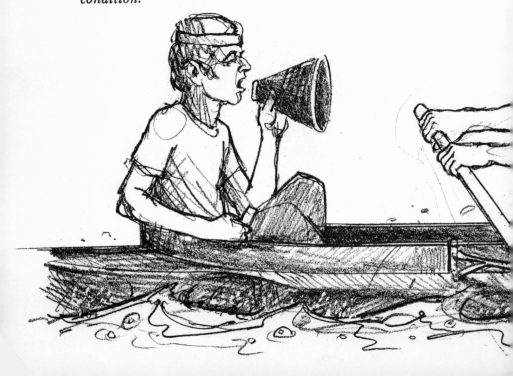

1928 that exercise which produced no discomfort helped digestion, and exercise which *did* simply delayed it.

Now, a word about jogging. It was originally recommended that it be done at a pace that would raise the heart rate to between 130 and 140 beats per minute. This, of course, automatically put it into the category of severe exercise, with all the complications and side effects I have mentioned.

I became very interested in the subject of jogging back in 1967 and put two researchers to work to study its effect in the Department of Experimental Surgery at McGill University. They ran mongrel dogs, two to five years of age and weighing 43 to 50 pounds, on a treadmill. The treadmill was set at a five-degree elevation, at 3 miles an hour, and the animals were run for 20 to 30 minutes a day. The speed and duration of exercise were gradually increased until the animals were running 5–7 miles an hour for 60 minutes. Our objective was to find out if this type of strenuous exercise would increase the collateral circulation of the animals' hearts, thus preventing them from dying if two of their coronary arteries were experimentally narrowed. After six weeks, we were amazed to find that two animals from the control group died suddenly, shortly after coming off the treadmill after a one-hour run (the control group animals did not have their coronary arteries narrowed).

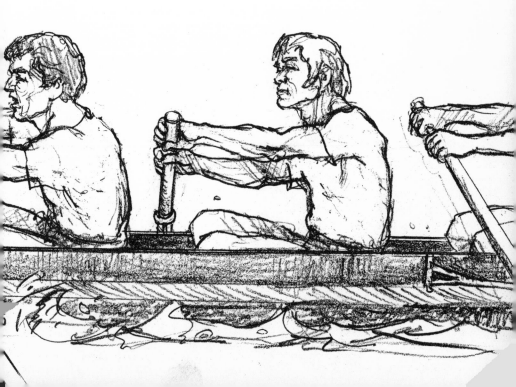

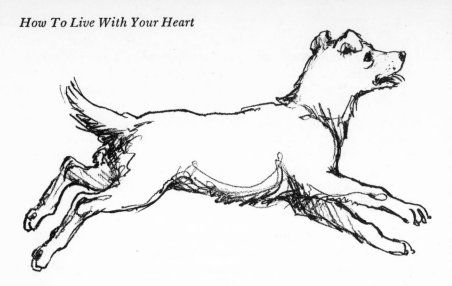

None of the exercised animals showed evidence that there had been development of collateral circulation in their hearts. The sudden deaths of 2 out of 14 animals with normal hearts who ran for a period of between six and seven weeks made us question the value of jogging.

We then proceeded to train another group of animals to jog for one hour a day for three months. At the end of that time, two out of three of their coronary arteries were narrowed by a mechanical constrictor. These animals showed no evidence that their three-month period of training had offered them any protection. After their chest wounds had healed, they were made to jog again. The result was that they died very suddenly of acute myocardial infarction—approximately one and a half times sooner than they might have died had they not been jogged.

On the basis of our experimental data, and from what I know of coronary artery disease, I do not believe that any patient should be subjected to severe jogging. Even if only one coronary artery is narrowed, a heart under the stress of jogging can go into sudden cardiac arrest. If there is disease of more than one artery, of course, the risk is increased.

There is a place for all kinds of exercise—even jogging. But the key word is moderation. Exercise that causes shortness of breath, or raises the pulse rate to high levels, is not to be recommended.

So much for classroom explanations. Now what are the basic dos and don'ts? What kind of exercise should you do, and what kind should you *not* do?

The table I have compiled (see p. 190) lists exercises which I think may be useful in your health program. It indicates the value of various exercises in terms of training the cardiovascular system at different ages. It also estimates the number of calories used up in the performance of different activities. It covers a wide range, from valueless calisthenics (valueless to the cardiovascular system) to extreme exertion activities such as mountain-climbing and crew racing. The basic advice, of course, is to practice common sense. My table provides the guidelines.

Perhaps the main point is that exercise should be *enjoyed*. If it can be done outdoors, all the better. Sun and fresh air can do wonders for people, whatever the activity.

I am a *walker* myself. I enjoy getting into comfortable clothing and going for a good hike several times a week. I try not to let the weather stop me. I therefore heartily recommend walking as an exercise for others. As a matter of fact, I believe that walking should be the basis of all exercise programs.

In addition to regular walking habits, everyone should engage in an hour of perspiration-generating exercise at least twice weekly. Although the average person is not conditioned for extreme running sessions, the system does need a certain amount of stress.

That hour, set aside twice weekly, may be used up in different ways—playing ball, swimming, perhaps just walking fast, with a little jogging thrown in for good measure. My own plan works well for many patients after revascularization surgery: walk 40 paces, jog 40 paces, walk 40 paces. Do this for an hour. Caution: for those who are overweight, or who have had revascularization surgery, the approach must be very gradual. It may take six months, or even a year, before a person is up to exercising for an hour.

In deciding on exercise plans, age must be considered—and 40 is usually a pretty good, if sometimes arbitrary, dividing line. I tell people all types of exercise are good if they are under 40, providing they have kept themselves fit. Overweight people who decide to start exercising again must be cautious. They should begin by simply walking. After 40, I urge people to slow down a little. I realize there are many men playing tennis singles after 40—but I also know there are a good many sudden deaths after severe exercise among those in the 40 to 60-year-old group.

The table at the back of the book spells out the value of different activities. But remember two points. First: to be truly beneficial, exercise must be done on a regular basis. Second: don't expect exercise to benefit your heart unless you also apply the principles of dieting discussed in the preceding chapter.

CHAPTER 8

Heart Surgery I
The Vineberg Procedure

Heart surgery has made some truly impressive strides in the last 25 years. Nonetheless, occasionally I lose sight of the fact and start complaining that things aren't developing fast enough. It is then that I run into someone like Adam K. and realize how far we've come.

Adam is 45 years old, looks more like a 60-year-old. He has come to me with a long history of *pressure* pain in the center of his chest. Occasionally the pain goes through to his back, between the shoulder blades. It comes after eating or exercise. He has pain in the arms, too, and shortness of breath even when he is not exerting himself. His heart *muscle* is not receiving an adequate supply of oxygenated blood. The cause: atherosclerosis of the major surface coronary arteries, a condition that narrows, and often blocks,

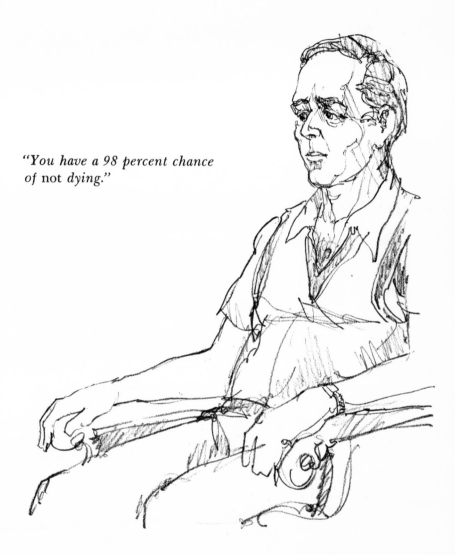

"You have a 98 percent chance of not *dying."*

the coronary arteries, thus preventing circulation of the blood to the heart.

On the advice of his doctor, he has agreed to the ultimate treatment—he has opted for surgery. There is no pretense as we sit talking. He is scared and doesn't mind showing it.

The conversation goes like this:

"*What are my chances of dying?*"

"*You have a 98 percent chance of not dying.*"

"*Will I be free of pain?*"

"*In your case, you have a 90 percent chance of having no pain, or certainly much less pain.*"

"*How long may I expect to live after the operation?*"

"*You have a 92 percent chance of being alive at the end of five years.*"

"*Will I be able to lead an active life?*"

"*Yes, you have an excellent chance of living an entirely normal life.*"

"*How long will the operation take?*"

"*Five hours, perhaps six.*" (The anesthetic alone may take as long as one hour to administer. A patient must be anesthetized slowly to avoid increasing his heart rate and to prevent the possibility of a sudden, and dangerous, drop in blood pressure.)

Adam, less frightened now, wants to know more about what happens after the operation. I tell him he'll be on his way home in three weeks after surgery, since he lives out of town. If he lived in Montreal, he would be allowed to go home after two weeks. I then explain that he will soon be able to walk, climb stairs, and return to work.

Then suddenly it hits me.

Adam is a very sick man, afraid one minute that he's going to die, and the next minute afraid that he won't. Not so many years ago, he would have been told to get his will and personal business in order. Today he is being told to make plans because he has an excellent chance, not only of surviving but of living a full, normal life.

This is not a surgeon's idle boast.

Among my patients are many whose operations date back 20 years or more. I have every reason to believe that when they die, it will be of some other cause, perhaps even plain old age. For those of us who practiced in the late 1930s, and even in the 1940s, the progress of surgery is nothing short of astounding. We have emerged from the dark ages of surgical science and we have done some incredible things.

I suppose it's only natural to think in personal terms and often, after an operation, my thoughts wander back to the mid-thirties and to my father, who had an acute myocardial infarction at the age of 53. How clearly I remember his terrible days and nights, the anguish and pain he suffered during the following five years.

He died in the prime of his life and there was nothing we could do for him then, except try to ease the pain. Today we might have saved his life.

Surgery has given new hope to the victims of heart disease. It has eclipsed the traditional medical treatment by drugs alone. But a word of caution: it is not the universal answer to coronary heart disease. Not everyone who has had a heart attack is a candidate for surgery. In some cases, surgical treatment is unnecessary. For instance, many people have attacks without ever being aware of them. (As mentioned earlier, attacks often are mistaken for bouts of indigestion.) The proof of this is that damage to the hearts of unsuspecting victims has shown up only after death when autopsies were ordered for other reasons.

How then does one select a case for surgery? My own rule of thumb is this:

A person with proven coronary artery disease with symptoms that persist more than one year should have his or her arteries studied by *cine coronary arteriography* (which provides a moving picture X ray of the arteries), to assess the seriousness of the condition. If this study shows diseased coronary arteries—one, two, or more of which are sufficiently blocked at their origins to cause his symptoms or endanger his life—the person should undergo surgery. One artery blocked $1\frac{1}{2}$–2 inches from its origin may not require surgery. Such an artery may form natural collaterals to bypass the point of occlusion. Thus a single artery narrowed along its course, particularly the right coronary artery with the main stem source undiseased, even with symptoms, may not require surgery. However, one artery blocked *at its origin* does require surgery. In my hospital, final decision is made jointly with cardiologist Dr. John Shanks and his colleagues who indicate when the surgery should be done—immediately or in a few months.

I have been preaching the benefits of heart surgery for most types of heart disease for a good many years now, with particular emphasis on cases of coronary heart disease. As I write this, I have many hundreds of patients who are proof of what I am talking about. They are people who, I believe, owe their lives to surgical treatment.

Unfortunately, there is still a considerable body of opposition to the idea of surgery. There is no doubt the opponents will some day come to accept the idea, but in the meantime, many people are dying unnecessarily.

I can understand the reluctance of patients to agree to surgery. There are people who have a very real fear of being put to sleep

NATURAL COLLATERALS

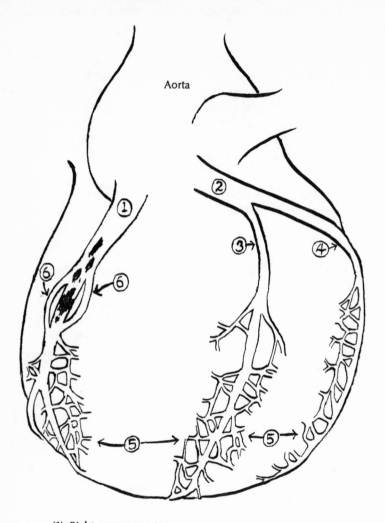

(1) Right coronary artery.

(2) Left coronary artery.

(3) Anterior descending artery.

(4) Circumflex artery.

(5) Myocardial arterioles.

(6) New branches of right coronary bypassing obstruction naturally.

Fig. 12. Natural collaterals may develop to relieve obstructions in distal surface coronary arteries.

and then not being able to wake up. Again, the surgeon himself is sometimes an object of fear. It is natural to resent someone poking around inside you with strange medical hardware.

I can forgive the layman but I find it hard indeed to follow the thinking of so many supposedly enlightened cardiologists who resist the idea of heart surgery. Certainly there are those who do recommend it, but there are altogether too many who don't, even when faced with a rather formidable array of statistics.

Then, too, there are the cardiologists who wait until their patients are in unmanageable condition before suggesting they visit a surgeon. The best medical (that is, nonsurgical) treatment of a coronary case can only be palliative. There is no medical cure. There are no known medical measures capable of restoring narrowed or blocked diseased coronary arteries to normal function. The problem, therefore, is one of simple hydraulics. Ways and means must be found to bring a new arterial supply of blood to the heart muscle through surgical intervention.

Let me try to explain the thinking of the cardiologists who oppose surgery. The rationalization is that heart surgery is still comparatively new and traditional concepts don't die easily. It wasn't all that long ago that a surgeon was considered to be doing the devil's work when he removed a person's appendix. The traditionalists proclaimed that God had placed the appendix in the human body for a *reason.*

In 1945, the year I returned from war service with the Canadian Medical Corps, the thought of doing anything at all for coronary heart disease—except for rest and medication—was ridiculed publicly. Performing heart surgery was regarded as lunacy of the first order.

True, some forward-looking surgeons had tried earlier to light up the immense darkness that surrounded the heart. Dr. C. S. Beck, of Western Reserve in Cleveland, was one. In 1935, he attempted to improve circulation to the left ventricle (one of the heart's large pumping chambers), by sewing a muscle graft to the surface of the heart. The attempt failed—muscle does not join with muscle too well. Two years later, Dr. L. O'Shaughnessy, working in England, tried to increase the arterial blood supply to the left ventricle by sewing a different type of graft to the ventricular muscle. This appeared to be partially successful, but unfortunately the work ended with O'Shaughnessy's untimely death on the beaches of Dunkirk during World War II.

There was a technique of heart catheterization, developed by Dr. Forssman in 1929 and taken up by Dr. Andre Cournand and

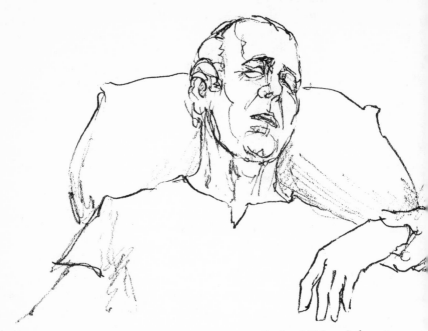

Dr. Dickinson Richards in 1941, by which holes in children's hearts could be shown in X rays. However, it was not until 1958 that Dr. Mason Sones and his team at the Cleveland Clinic, developed cine coronary *arteriograms* for visualization of each coronary artery. Prior to this, the only way to know the true condition of the coronary artery pipelines, their branches, communications among each other, and outside arterial communication with the heart, was to wait until the patient died. Only examination on the autopsy table yielded this information.

The fact is that the final chapter always unfolds in the pathologist's laboratory. Only by studying thousands of hearts on the autopsy table can you learn anything about a disease. Yet the vast majority of cardiologists rarely saw the inside of an autopsy room after leaving medical school. There were some exceptions, one of them being Dr. P. M. Zoll, a cardiologist at Beth Israel Hospital in Boston, who worked with pathologist Dr. M. J. Schlesinger. Dr. Zoll correlated his pathological studies very closely with his clinical findings.

The cardiologist of the 1950s talked about dye tests which measure how much blood the heart pumps per minute. They read

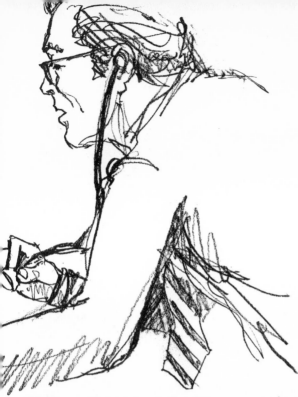

Many cardiologists of the 50's were against surgery; they sat by the patient's bed while he died.

electrocardiograms but they didn't know the pathological anatomy of the human heart, or of the coronary arteries, except in a general way. They were too busy to go to the autopsy room.

The average cardiologist believed the patient could get along better *without* surgery. He sat by the patient's bedside while he died, reassuring the family, of course, that everything possible had been done. His knowledge of the disease was based upon the patient's complaints of pain, his ability to exercise on the two-step, and multiple electrocardiograms which at that time were extremely inaccurate. Among other things, cardiologists thought that with a diminished blood supply, the heart would form new collateral channels to accommodate the flow of blood and thus alleviate the crisis.

The idea was pretty hard to follow. What they were saying was that in some mysterious way, blood would come from outside the heart to join the heart muscle when the coronary artery was blocked. It was, you might say, asking a lot, particularly when pathologists such as Dr. Schlesinger proved through special injection studies of many human hearts that this rarely happened.

115

The only time extracardiac blood channels may occur is after a myocardial infarction, when the scarred heart muscle and pericardium, (the sac that holds the heart) fuse together. The blood vessels may then come through the pericardium right into the heart. This occurs rarely and when it does, it forms an extracoronary blood supply. For the most part, however, the heart is suspended in its sac, isolated from the rest of the circulation. It is completely dependent on its coronary artery pipelines for oxygenated blood for its contracting muscles.

Stages Leading to the Vineberg Operation

Before World War II, when I was teaching anatomy and removing lungs, I often stopped to examine the internal mammary arteries lying there and thought, "If only I could get them into the heart." They looked ideal. These two arteries lie beneath the breast bone (sternum), supplying it, the chest muscles, and breasts with oxygenated blood. They are about the same size as a coronary artery and can be safely separated from the underside of the breast bone, without endangering the blood supply to the breast or chest muscles. They are present in both sexes, but are larger in the male.

I was convinced that if you wanted to get more blood into the heart, it couldn't be through the diseased surface coronary arteries. Let me put it this way: a house has a country water system. When the tap stops working, the owner calls the plumber who digs down five feet and finds the pipe blocked. He puts a new piece in the pipe but the following summer the tap goes dry again because the pipe becomes blocked further down. This pretty well sums up the pathology of coronary artery disease.

Coronary atherosclerosis usually involves the coronary artery pipelines in many places in a disseminated manner, just as the rust involves the water pipe in more than one place. It is for this reason that, like a good plumber, I believe it's necessary to lay in a completely new pipeline that does not rust, rather than repair the old one.

With this thought in mind, I started my experiments with the implantation of mammary arteries into the hearts of animals. These led to what was considered a major breakthrough in the treatment of coronary artery disease—at least in animals. There were the skeptics. "It might work in animals," they said. "But, on humans . . .?" I ignored the skepticism, being certain we were on the right track, one leading to a possible revolution in the treatment.

LEFT VENTRICULAR INTERNAL MAMMARY
ARTERY IMPLANT

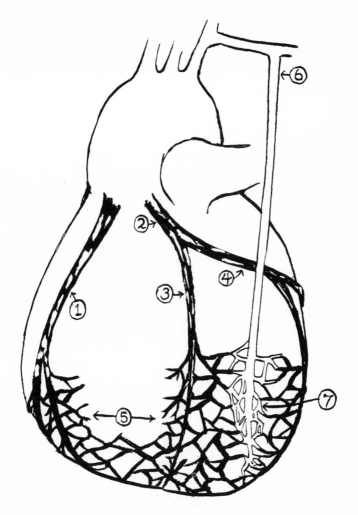

Fig. 13. (1) Diseased right coronary artery

(2) Diseased left coronary artery

(3) Diseased anterior descending coronary artery

(4) Diseased circumflex artery

(5) Non-diseased myocardial arterioles

(6) Non-diseased left internal mammary artery

(7) New branches of mammary artery implanted in heart muscle.

117

In the Vineberg operations, the diseased conorary arteries and their surface branches (the old rusty pipelines), which are supplying enough oxygenated blood to the heart to keep the patient living, are not touched. Instead, new arterial lines are set up in the heart muscle, bypassing all occluded surface coronary arteries. These new arterial pipelines supply the heart with a new source of oxygenated blood. I have developed five such operations. Revascularization operation No. 1, the original Vineberg Operation, concerned the implantation of the left internal mammary artery into the left ventricular wall.

The technique took five years to develop in the experimental laboratory, and was first used to revascularize human hearts in 1950. In this operation, the left internal mammary artery, which originates as a branch of the main artery to the arm (subclavian) and ends in the muscle of the abdomen, is carefully teased away from the undersurface of the chest bone for a distance of 8–9 inches, and all its branches which supply the chest muscles are tied. The internal mammary artery is disconnected where it enters the abdominal muscle. (Fig. 3). This completely removes it from its normal location, except for its attachment to the artery going to the arm from which it gets its blood supply. The sac that contains the heart (the pericardium) is split open, exposing all four heart pumps.

A tunnel is made in the muscular wall of the left ventricle for left implants and in that of the right ventricle for right implants. The tunnel is usually 1½–2 inches long. (Fig. 4). In the left ventricle, it is placed deep between the termination of the branches of the surface coronary arteries. The free portion of the internal mammary artery is pulled into the tunnel with one to three side branches cut open to allow free bleeding into the myocardial sinusoidal spaces. This removes the blood and helps keep the artery open. (Fig. 20). The closed end of the artery is fixed to the heart muscle at the end of the tunnel with a cotton suture. The other end is left connected to the large artery supplying blood to the arm. In this way, arterial blood escapes from the artery through its open side branches into the tunnel in the left ventricular myocardium. (Fig. 21). The contracting action of the heart carries the blood away and helps to keep the artery open. At the end of twelve days, the implanted internal mammary artery starts to send out true arterial branches. (Fig. 19). These branches grow and seek out other smaller arteries in the myocardium, which are the terminal branches of the surface coronary arteries. The new branches join

118

with the terminal branches of the surface coronary arteries in six weeks to two months after implantation to supply the myocardium originally supplied by the diseased surface coronary arteries. (Fig. 13).

Anatomically, in 72 percent of patients in whom this occurs, it is possible for one internal mammary artery to supply oxygenated blood to the terminal branches of all three coronary arteries, via the nondiseased myocardial arteriolar networks, when all the patient's own coronary arteries are blocked. An internal mammary artery thus implanted into the left ventricular wall acts as a new pipeline, bypassing diseased surface coronary arteries, to carry fresh oxygenated blood to the contracting heart muscle via the non-diseased intramyocardial arterioles.

In 1950 a Finnish tailor came to me on the advice of his doctor who had read about my experimental work in the newspapers. This man was in poor shape indeed. His heart was so bad, in fact, that he hadn't been out of his room for two years.

I operated on him but his blood pressure remained very low during surgery. I wanted to use a vasopressor, an agent that raises blood pressure, which I had seen Dr. Reginald Smithwick, of the Massachusetts General Hospital in Boston, use on patients with hypertension. However, our cardiologists said that the vasopressor would constrict the coronary arteries and that if I used it, I'd kill my patient. A ridiculous statement, I thought, because how could hard, stiff diseased coronary arteries be constricted by a vasopressor drug.

I didn't use a vasopressor on the tailor and he was dead 62 hours after he went on the operating table. Then at autopsy, we made an interesting discovery: only one coronary artery with a lumen the size of a pin head was open in his entire heart at the time of surgery. In other words, his coronary arteries had become almost totally useless. He died because this, the only patent artery in his heart, became blocked with a fresh clot. The internal mammary artery I had implanted in the heart, however, was wide open and there was no clot. Unfortunately, the patient hadn't lived long enough for the implanted internal mammary artery to branch and supply the heart with fresh oxygenated blood. The patient had died—but in a very real sense, the operation had been a success.

"What can you expect when you operate on a patient with coronary artery disease?" a cardiologist shrugged. Better results, I said to myself. And I was determined to press on. From that time on, I used a vasopressor. Today, cardiologists all over the

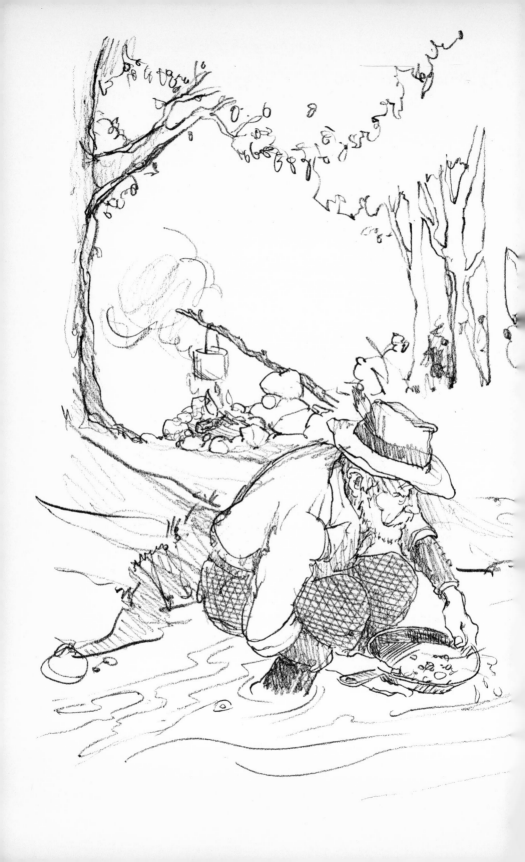

world use vasopressor drugs to keep blood pressures up in patients with myocardial infarction due to coronary artery disease. They are used daily in coronary care units.

Then along came my second patient, a prospector from the West. He knew my first patient had died, but he also knew he was pretty near the end of the line himself and was ready to take any risk.

I liked Henry. He was gutsy, a real great fellow—and at 54 severely disabled. When he arrived he actually was suffering heart failure, and the condition worsened on the operating table. I worked quickly and hoped for the best. After he came out of anesthesia, he did well. Three weeks later, he was on a westbound plane. Five month later, he was back prospecting. He lived and worked pain-free for more than 10 years after surgery.

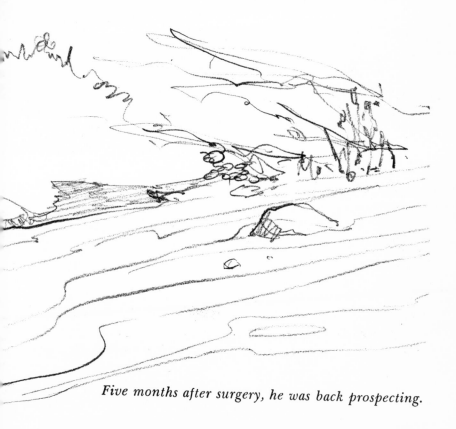

Five months after surgery, he was back prospecting.

The operation has been a success and people began taking me seriously. In 1952, the late Dr. Walter Scriver, then professor of medicine, set up a medical team to work with me at the Royal Victoria Hospital. It included Dr. Phillip Hill, Dr. Peter Pare and later, Dr. John Shanks. I might stress here that it's important for a surgeon to work in conjunction with one or two cardiologists. Over the years, I have always relied on a cardiologist to determine whether a patient truly has coronary artery disease, and if so, whether he needs surgery. The cardiologist prepares the patient for surgery, comes into the operating room from time to time, and joins me in following him through the postoperative period. If the person lives out of town, his own cardiologist is advised about postoperative care. If he lives in Montreal, he is followed up by our cardiologist.

The cardiologists with whom I have worked were thoroughly familiar with the anatomy and pathology of coronary artery circulation. They also know, from many years of experience with me, how much surgery a patient can tolerate. Great care is given to the selection and medical treatment of my patients, a fact which accounts for our very low mortality. It's no accident that we are able to handle people who have been rejected in other centers. (I would also commend those experienced, highly-specialized anesthetists who administer only to heart patients. They, too, have played a major role in our success with patients in the bad risk category. And we have had many of them.)

By 1958 we had begun to table the statistical evidence. Of forty patients whose angina had not been decubitus (that is, they suffered no pain at rest) and who had been followed up to six years postoperatively, 28 had slight or no angina and one had considerably less pain. This was an improvement rate of 73 percent, not bad for a start.

The results were less satisfactory for patients with angina decubitus. This type of patient was not operated upon again until 1962 when I had developed the rapidly acting epicardiectomy and free omental graft to supplement implants (these will be explained later in this chapter).

The operations continued. One satisfied patient referred another. Doctors with satisfied patients sent others. It was a snowball effect and our unit was well on its way to success. For me, it was a very busy time because, in addition to performing a great many operations, I was also lecturing and presenting new data to meetings all over the world.

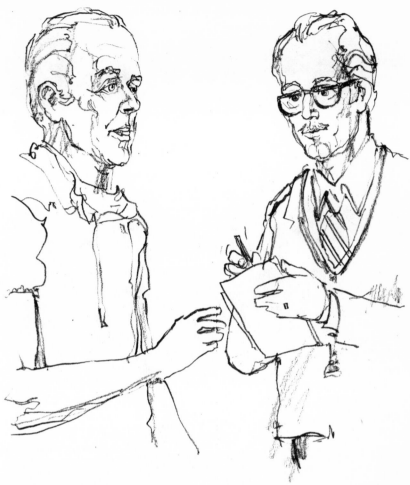

It's important for a surgeon to work in conjunction with a cardiologist.

There was still skepticism, of course. The Cleveland Clinic, for instance, doubted that the internal mammary arteries I had implanted could still be open. I took up the challenge. In November, 1961, I sent a patient to Dr. Mason Sones, so that he could see for himself. He agreed to study his arteries and report back.

Then one day the telephone rang in my office. It was Dr. Sones in Cleveland. He was so excited, he was shouting and I had to hold the receiver away from my ear. He had completed his study and

123

ARTERIAL PHOTOGRAPH

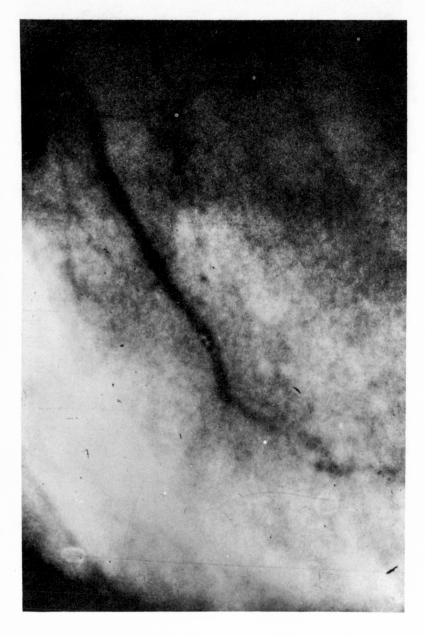

Fig. 14. Photo taken from a cine angiogram by Dr. Sones of an implanted internal mammary artery. This is seven and a half years after surgery. The functioning implanted artery is seen in the center supplying blood to the heart muscle.

was satisfied that the internal mammary artery I had implanted $7\frac{1}{2}$ years before was indeed wide open, and supplying oxygenated blood to the heart. (Fig. 14). The patient's right and left main coronary arteries were markedly narrowed. (Fig. 15). Five years later the patient died following surgery. At autopsy his right and left coronary arteries were completely blocked. Injection of the $12\frac{1}{2}$-year-old mammary artery implant with radio-opaque mass showed filling of the entire coronary arterial system up to their areas of occlusion. Histopathological sections of the implanted internal mammary artery showed it fully patent without disease. (Fig. 16). The implanted internal mammary artery was the only artery supplying oxygenated blood to the patient's heart.

Dr. Sones sent his associate, Dr. Donald Effler, head of chest surgery, to Montreal to watch me operate and learn the technique of implanting the left internal mammary artery into the wall of the left ventricle. Dr. Effler paid three visits to our hospital and con-

ANGIOGRAM OF LEFT CORONARY SYSTEM

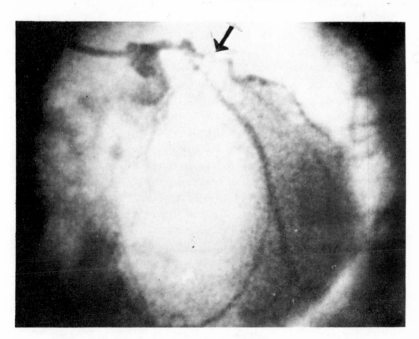

Fig. 15. Cine coronary angiogram showing disease of the left, anterior descending and circumflex coronary arteries seven and a half years after left ventricular mammary implant shown in preceding photograph.

cluded that the operation was a milestone in heart surgery. He started doing implant operations in Cleveland soon after and had so much faith in the procedure that he christened it the *Vineberg Implant Operation.* From that time to date Dr. Effler has been a strong supporter of mammary artery ventricular implants for the treatment of diffuse coronary artery atherosclerosis. Wide-scale implant surgery was now on its way.

Every operation brought fresh evidence that mammary artery implants were working. There was the chef I operated on in 1953, for example. He didn't get better after surgery and took a sedentary job as a parking lot attendant. This was a disappointment to me. Three and a half years later he underwent a second operation, this one performed by a Denver surgeon, who found a huge aneurysm, or bulge, in the wall of the right ventricle which had not been present in the earlier operation in Montreal.

The patient died from it on the operating table and an autopsy was performed. The report showed the only artery open in the heart was the mammary artery implant I had placed there three and a half years before. It was supplying blood to the left ventricle where it had been implanted, but obviously not to the right ventricle since it developed an aneurysm. When he came to me originally for surgery, at least one of his own coronary arteries must have been open, or else he never would have survived the operation. After the operation, however, progressive atherosclerosis completely closed all of his coronary arteries, so that he was living on the internal mammary artery which I had implanted. The latter, unlike his own coronary arteries, had not developed atherosclerosis.

MICROPHOTOGRAPH

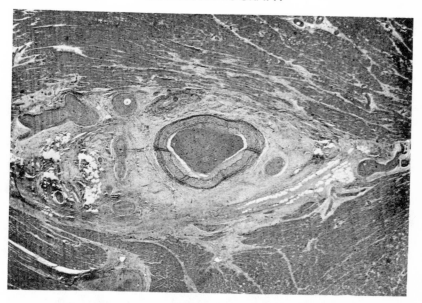

Fig. 16. This microphotograph shows a mammary artery twelve and a half years after left ventricular implant. It was the only artery open in this patient's heart.

OPERATION NO. 3

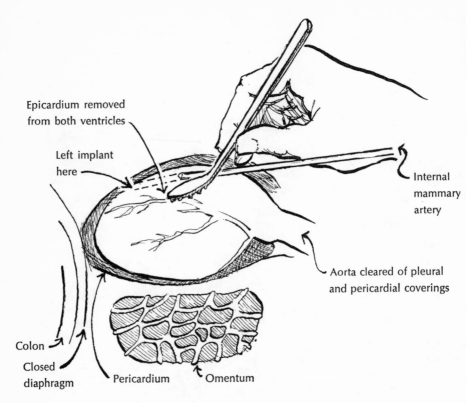

Epicardium removed
from both ventricles

Left implant
here

Internal
mammary
artery

Aorta cleared of pleural
and pericardial coverings

Colon

Closed
diaphragm

Pericardium

Omentum

Fig. 17. A left ventricular internal mammary artery implant with
epicardiectomy and free omental graft.

Further Development of the Vineberg Operation

The operations had been revolutionary, but it was now becoming clear that we would have to do more than implant one artery if we were to save more lives. We needed to find the means of distributing the blood of an internal mammary artery from one point to another. We then developed *epicardiectomy,* which is the surgical removal of the serous layer of the pericardium (the tissue which covers the coronary vessels and heart muscle). This technique is used to open collateral channels in the left ventricle, (Fig. 17), and it was added to what was becoming widely known as the *Vineberg procedure.* Later we used a free omental graft to carry blood from one place to another and to channel fresh arterial blood

OPERATION NO. 3

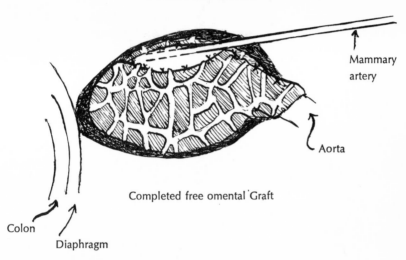

Mammary
artery

Aorta

Completed free omental Graft

Colon

Diaphragm

Fig. 18. Completed left ventricular internal mammary artery implant with epicardiectomy and free omental graft.

from the pericardial sac vessels into the coronary arteries. This was revascularization operation No. 2.

In this operation the greater omentum (the fatty apron lying in the abdomen) is removed from the bowel to which it is attached. In so doing all of its blood supply is cut off. This piece of primitive tissue, however, quickly obtains a new blood supply. It stimulates vessels in contact with both of its surfaces to grow into it from the vascular pericardial sac and from the underlying coronary arteries. The serous layer of the pericardium is surgically removed and the epicardium covering the heart muscle and coronary artery is likewise removed. Thus when placed around the heart, vessels grow into it from the pericardial vessels and from the coronary vessels. In this way oxygenated blood is poured into its networks from the pericardial vessels to enter the underlying coronary arteries and heart muscle, thus bypassing many areas of coronary artery disease. After three years of testing in the laboratory, the operation was used in the treatment of human coronary artery disease.

129

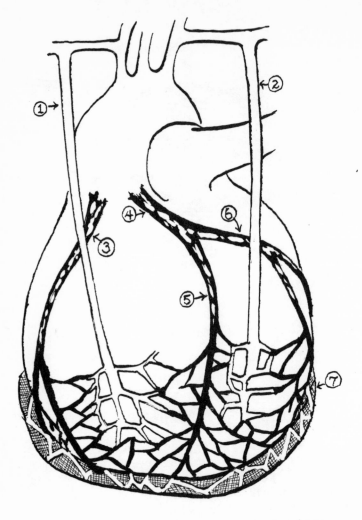

(1) Non-diseased right internal mammary artery implanted into right ventricular wall.

(2) Non-diseased left internal mammary artery implanted into left ventricular wall.

(3, 4, 5, 6) Diseased coronary arteries.

(7) Free omental graft.

Fig. 19. Right and left ventricular internal mammary artery implants with epicardiectomy and free omental graft.

This operation was used on many patients in conjunction with single and later with double internal mammary artery implants. A variation of this operation became my revascularization operation No. 3. (Figs. 17, 18).

In this operation the epicardium over individual large surface coronary arteries is split and spread to either side exposing many fine vessels in the pericoronary fat. A piece of omentum 1 inch wide, containing two to three blood vessels is fashioned in the form of a strip and sutured to the reflected epicardium so that the omental strip lies directly on the diseased coronary artery for its entire length. It is fixed to the pulmonary artery, or to the aorta, at its upper end. In both the free omental graft operations, the omentum stimulates blood vessels to grow into both of its surfaces, allowing oxygenated blood to flow from the pericardium and other large vessels into it and then into the underlying coronary artery.

As our work progressed, mortality rates dropped to almost zero. At one point, I had done 54 implants without a single death. However, some of my patients began coming back with pain. We had successfully done left ventricular mammary artery implants and these were still open. But cine coronary arteriography showed that our patients with recurring or persistent pain also had diseased right coronary arteries. This led to revascularization operation No. 4, in which the right internal mammary artery is implanted into the right ventricular wall.

This was a special technique because the wall of the right ventricle is only one-fifth of an inch thick and the tunnel is thus difficult to make. I have been successful with these implants. However, they cannot be done when the right ventricular muscle has been replaced by fat, a condition which occasionally occurs in patients over 65 years of age.

Revascularization operation No. 5 was the ultimate combination technique in which right and left internal mammary arteries were implanted into right and left ventricular walls in the same operation. (Fig. 19). The procedure was carried out on a large series of patients with success. The use of the two arteries has been necessary for those patients that by cine coronary arteriography

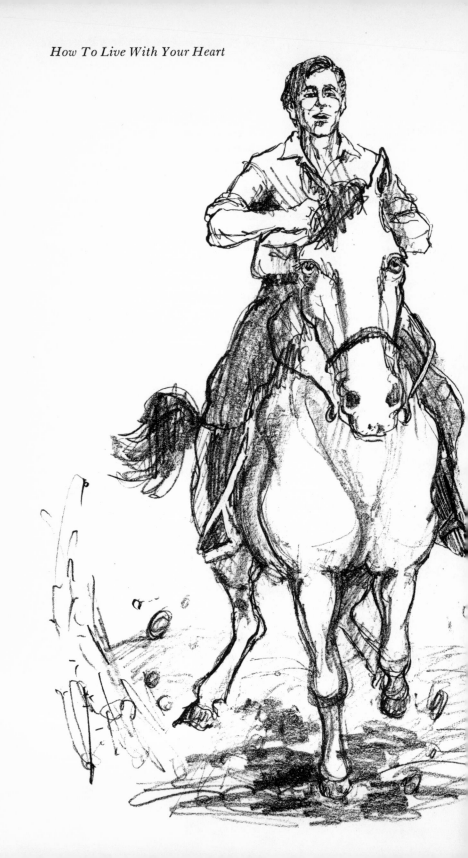

show disease of the right coronary artery as well as the anterior descending and circumflex coronary arteries of the left side. Years before, many patients had had a left internal mammary artery implanted in the wall of the left ventricle. This implant was functioning well, but the patient's own coronary arteries had become so completely obstructed that a second artery was needed.

Internal mammary artery implants have proven themselves over and over through the years. Cine coronary arteriography and pathological injection studies frequently reveal that these are the only arteries supplying oxygenated blood to the heart of patients. For some reason we do not yet understand, the internal mammary artery does not develop atherosclerosis either in its original location beneath the chest bone, or after it has been implanted in the human ventricular heart wall.

After surgery, many patients have gone on to lead normal active lives.

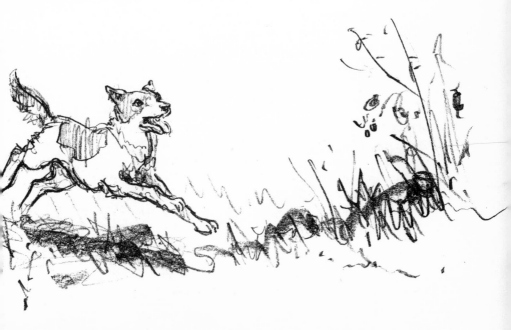

CHAPTER 9

Heart Surgery II
Revascularization and Other Procedures

From the start we had been trying to find a way to revascularize the entire heart, so that even if all the coronary arteries became blocked, the heart itself would continue to function.

We think we have accomplished this by the combined operations of right and left ventricular internal mammary artery implants, complemented by the supplementary operations of epicardiectomy and free omental grafts.

Our long-term studies, over twenty-four years, showed that the implanted internal mammary arteries were capable of maintaining human hearts when all of the patient's own coronary arteries had become completely blocked. This confirmed that our objective—revascularization of the entire heart—had been reached.

Our statistics offered great hope for very sick heart patients. For example, of a particular group of 76 cases with chronic left ventricular heart failure treated by implant surgery, there was a 10 percent operative mortality rate and an 85 percent rate of marked improvement over 3.2 years. After an average interval of 4.5 years, 49 percent of the patients were still living.

This was most rewarding, because patients with chronic left ventricular failure due to extensive coronary artery obstructions had (and still have) a very poor prognosis for the future. I maintain that patients who, after multiple heart attacks, still have 50 percent of their left ventricular muscle living and unscarred, can be helped by ventricular internal mammary artery implants. These supply oxygenated blood to the unscarred but ischemic muscle through which the patient is living. Our experience has proven this to be true.

Evidence that revascularization by internal mammary artery implants prolongs life is shown by another recently studied group of 48 patients who had undergone simultaneous right and left implants. In all cases, there was cine angiographic evidence of extensive main-stem coronary artery disease. Forty-two of these patients were considered very advanced cases, having had triple to quadruple main-stem coronary artery disease. There was one (or 2.1 percent) operative death among them. Anginal pain was relieved in 90 percent of the patients, and, in 75 percent of those with failure, chronic left ventricular failure was relieved. Forty of the patients had already had at least one heart attack before their operations.

If they had been treated medically, 20 of the group (or 42 percent) would have been dead at the end of five years, according to published medical statistics. In our series there were only three late deaths. After five years, the total mortality (both operative and late) was four patients (or 8 percent); 44 patients (or 92 percent) were still alive. Our revascularization experience with ventricular arterial implants and supplementary procedures at this writing includes 680 patients—among them quite a few 20-year survivors.

Internal mammary artery implants have definite advantages. For one thing, they do not develop atherosclerosis. As least 87 percent of them remain open in the human heart muscle for many, many years. They supply blood to the myocardial arterioles, which do not become diseased. They have been proven to be the only arteries supplying oxygenated blood to a human heart when atherosclerosis has closed all of a patient's own arteries. The operation can be performed with less than 2 percent operative loss and with an overall improvement of 70—90 percent. It is beneficial in the treatment of patients with chronic heart failure and is ideal for those with extensive disseminated coronary atherosclerosis. It

135

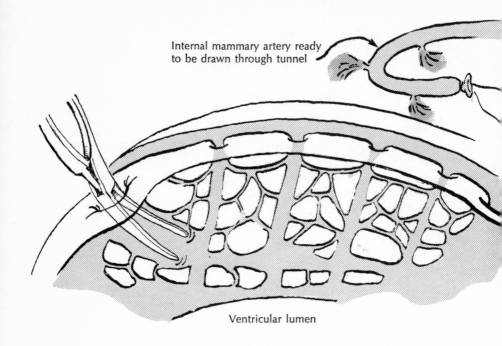

Fig. 20. A blunt forceps is used to create a tunnel in the heart muscle through which the bleeding internal mammary artery will be drawn.

has been shown to supply up to 150 cc. per minute of fresh oxygenated blood from one to four years after implantation. It can be used to revascularize left ventricle heart muscle even when half of that muscle has been solidly scarred by previous heart attacks.

The implants, of course, have their disadvantages as well. For example, they take time to branch, and except in the case of the

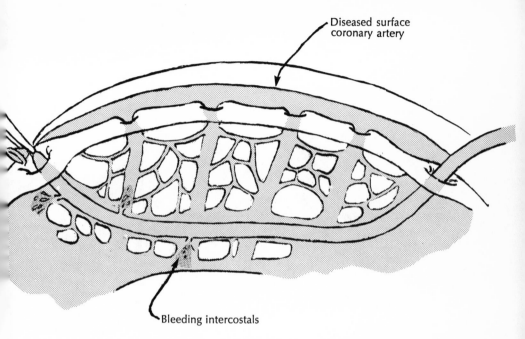

Diseased surface
coronary artery

Bleeding intercostals

Fig. 21. Internal mammary artery, bleeding freely into tunnel
and myocardial sinusoids.

right ventricular implant, the benefit to the patient is not immediate. They can't be used where there are many islands of scar in
the left ventricular muscle and when the left ventricular wall is
very thin. Again, they can't be used for immediate revascularization in the treatment of an impending heart attack.

Pericoronary omental strip grafts also have their advantages

AORTO CORONARY VEIN GRAFT BY-PASS

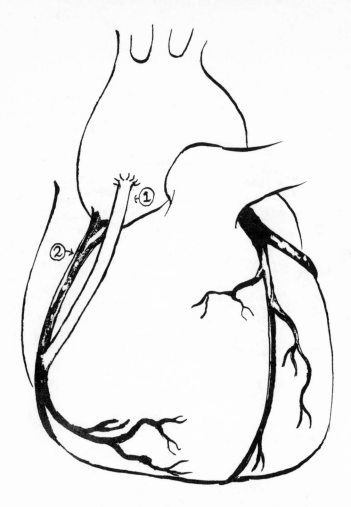

Fig. 22. The blocked right coronary artery is revascularized.
(1) Vein by-pass. (2) Right coronary artery.

and disadvantages. On the one hand is the fact that they form an arteriolar circulation within eight days. On the other hand, it happens that sometimes the greater omentum is not fit for use. It may be scarred, or too fat. Furthermore, sometimes it is congenitally absent.

138

The Aorta Coronary Vein Bypass Graft

While I was refining the Vineberg procedure, others were devising different means of alleviating the disease through direct repair of arteries.

One of these procedures was endarterectomy, an operation to reopen blocked coronary arteries by scraping out the substances blocking their insides. This is similar to scraping out the rust in a galvanized iron water pipe.

Another was the aorta-coronary vein bypass graft. In this operation, a vein is taken from the thigh. One end is sewn to the edges of a hole made in the large aorta (the biggest artery in the body) leaving the left ventricle. The other end is sewn to the edges of a hole made in the blocked coronary artery beyond the point where it is obstructed. Oxygenated blood pours from the great aorta into the vein graft and thus into the coronary artery. This is called a bypass operation because a vein is used to bypass the blockage in an artery or arteries. Three or more grafts are needed when all three coronary arteries are diseased. (Fig. 23).

Aorto-coronary vein bypass operations have many advantages. For example, they supply oxygenated blood immediately to a coronary artery beyond the point of obstruction in large quantities. Again, because the grafts work immediately, the period of convalescence is shortened. They are ideal for the treatment of proximal localized coronary artery disease in younger patients. These operations are also performed to prevent myocardial infarction in patients in whom it appears about to occur. Their use in the treatment of these patients seems worthwhile.

However, the use of aorto-coronary vein bypass grafts for patients who have had acute infarction and who are not doing well medically has not been too satisfactory. In many centers, in fact, the treatment of the acute myocardial infarction by aorto-coronary vein bypass grafts has been discontinued. Recent published data indicate that, for patients who had an acute myocardial infarction within two months preceding the operation, there is a 14.5 percent operative mortality following aorto-coronary vein bypass grafts. In addition, there are reports that patients develop acute myocardial infarction following aorto-coronary vein bypass grafts. The percentage differs according to the center reporting and ranges from 4 to 25 percent. Thus it is too early to be sure of the value of these grafts in treating patients with recent myocardial infarctions as compared with standard medical treatment. The procedure

TRIPLE AORTO-CORONARY VEIN BYPASS
OPERATION

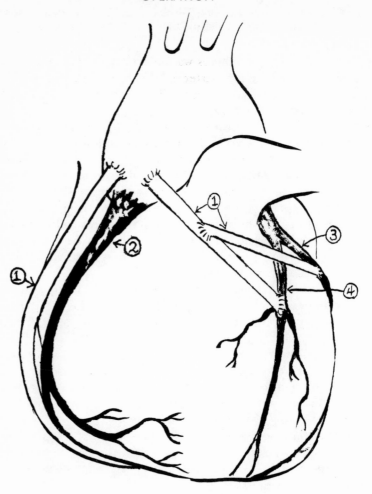

Fig. 23. (1) Vein bypass.

(2) Slightly-diseased right coronary artery.

(3) Diseased circumflex coronary artery.

(4) Diseased anterior descending coronary artery.

INTERNAL MAMMARY ARTERY CORONARY ARTERY BYPASS

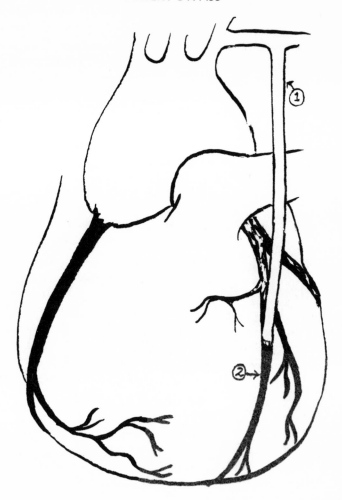

Fig. 24. Internal mammary artery (1) joined to cut end of coronary artery (2) as practiced by many surgeons.

seems worthwhile in desperate situations, provided patients are in well-equipped centers with experienced personnel.

Certainly one fact supports the aorto-coronary vein bypass procedure as a treatment, namely its apparent success with the pre-infarction and possibly the acute infarction state, particularly in patients who can't be helped by any other operative procedure. It is our experience with internal mammary artery implants used to treat chronic myocardial ischemia, that they take too long to work to be of benefit in the acute infarction state.

Recently we have found that an internal mammary artery implanted into a six-hour-old acute myocardial infarction by a new technique supplies oxygenated blood to the muscle in the area of infarction immediately, thus saving the heart muscle. This operative procedure is in its preliminary stages, having been performed only on animals. However, it soon should be ready for human usage.

Let us consider for a moment the disadvantages of aorto-coronary vein bypass grafts. To start with, open heart surgery is necessary to do these grafts, adding an extra risk to the operation. Moreover, of patients with coronary artery disease, at least 44 percent, according to pathological studies, have disease in the second part of surface coronary arteries. This may not be detected by cine coronary arteriography in the living, contracting human heart. Such disease thus may be present beyond the point at which the bypass graft has been attached. In such cases, the fresh oxygenated blood pours into vessels whose disease is not detected by cine coronary arteriography.

In addition vein grafts pour oxygenated blood into the second half of coronary arteries thus bypassing heart muscle supplied by branches from the first half of the coronary arteries. It is similar to supplying the State of New York with fresh water from a Vermont Lake using pipelines which go directly to Manhattan Island without branches to the rest of the state. The excess water goes into the ocean, just as the excess blood goes out through the coronary veins (sinus). Pipelines buried in the soil with branches, like internal mammary arteries, supply the entire state. The same is true of the operation of Dr. George E. Green of St. Luke's Hospital in New York City. Dr. Green sutures the open end of an internal mammary artery, after it has been separated from the sternum and cut away from its abdominal attachments, directly to a coronary artery beyond its point of occlusion. Like the aortocoronary vein bypass graft, it pours oxygenated blood into coronary arteries which may be diseased beyond their points of obstruction. The Green operation of internal mammary artery to coronary artery anastomose is not to be confused with the Vineberg internal mammary artery implant procedure.

Between 22 and 24 percent of all vein grafts performed on humans are said to block within a year, and 30 percent at the end of two years. This is probably not due to technical problems but rather to turbulence that sometimes develops in the blood coursing through the coronary artery. The problem may also stem from the undetected disease in the coronary artery beyond the vein graft. Furthermore, in a considerable number of cases, when a vein graft blocks, the artery to which it is attached may also block, thus preventing replacement with another vein graft. In such cases I have implanted internal mammary arteries with good results.

The grafts have not been successful in reversing chronic left ventricular failure. Also, patients who have had previous heart attacks do not do as well as those whose hearts have not been scarred by previous attacks.

It is too early to give a long-term prognosis for initially successful cases. Bypass grafts have been performed for only five years.

The Vineberg procedure also has disadvantages, one of which is that left internal mammary artery implants take from two to six months to grow branches large enough to supply the heart muscle with adequate oxygenated blood. (Actually, most patients show improvement at the end of six months.)

On the other hand, there are these advantages:

Internal mammary arteries do not become diseased. They have been shown to remain open and functioning for at least $17\frac{1}{2}$ years.

One implant placed in the proper position has a 72 percent chance of revascularizing the whole heart. It has been shown by cine angiography, as well as at autopsy, that one implanted internal mammary artery keeps patients alive and well when progressive atherosclerosis has closed all or most of his own coronary arteries.

Open heart surgery with its complications is not necessary in implant surgery.

Even when an implant does not perform as expected, it does no harm. The internal mammary arteries in the Vineberg procedure are implanted into heart muscle between coronary arteries. Thus, unlike a vein graft which blocks, if the artery should block, it does not cause a blockage of any coronary artery. The implant operation in no way interferes with the coronary arteries upon which the patient is living when he comes to surgery. If necessary, another artery may be implanted into the heart muscle alongside the blocked mammary artery.

There are quite a few surgeons in North America and Western Europe who are having success with left ventricular internal mammary artery implants. However, many of them immediately modified the operation. These have not been successful and have been abandoned for the newer procedure of aorto-coronary vein bypass grafts. There are many reasons why those who have failed to follow our technique do not have permanently open internal mammary artery implants. One is that they haven't taken the time to visit those surgeons who have had successful implants, to learn the technique properly. In the hands of those who have not really studied details of the implant procedure, it would appear that the operative mortality is too high, the complications too numerous, and the results poor.

Preoperative Examination of Patient

The operative mortality from any form of revascularization surgery depends upon many factors, one of which is the preoperative screening for noncardiac conditions that may influence the course of the patient during and after surgery. In my service, patients are given complete, thorough checkups. We particularly look for sources of chronic infection such as infected sinuses, teeth, urinary, and genital tracts. An overlooked abscessed tooth may result in heart failure when the patient is given an anesthetic. Special tests for emphysema are done, particularly in patients with large round chests—good lungs are essential for recovery from heart surgery of any type. Possible disease of the gallbladder must be known in case abdominal pain develops after surgery. The presence of a peptic ulcer presents the possibility of bleeding after surgery. This is a hazard unless recognized and treated before, during, and after surgery. Allergies to drugs may cause serious drops in blood pressure during and after the operation. Because of the character of coronary artery atherosclerosis, for a number of years I have anticoagulated my patients—that is, put them on blood thinners prior to surgery. This treatment is continued during and after surgery. We believe this helps prevent clotting in ragged coronary arteries, clotting which may cause myocardial infarction and possible death.

Cine coronary arteriography carries certain complications. Patients who have had it should not undergo major surgery for at least 10 days to two weeks after the catheterization has been performed, in case a complication from the catheterization shows itself during

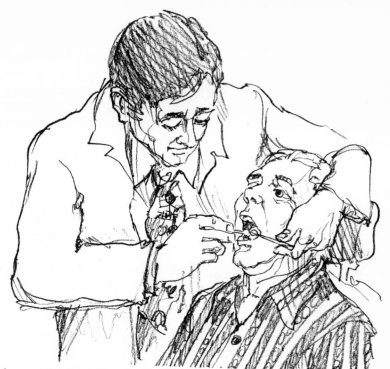

An overlooked abscessed tooth may result in heart failure under anesthia.

or after surgery. These are just a few of the many conditions which may influence the results in any form of revascularization surgery.

In 1950 I asked the late Dr. Lyman Duff, professor of pathology at McGill University what kind of patients I should operate on. He answered, "Arthur, let me tell you what type of cases you should not operate upon. You do not operate upon patients who have had a recent myocardial infarction. You should wait at least six months." I asked, "Why not?" Dr. Duff replied, "The infarcted muscle heals by scar and no scar is firm anywhere in the body under six months." He pointed out that a cut over a boxer's eye tends to reopen if the fighter goes back into the ring too soon. In the human heart new scar from a fresh infarction may stretch when the heart is stressed by surgery. This may result in heart failure on the operating table, or in possible progression of the infarction.

During the past 24 years we have postponed surgery in all of our patients for six months after an acute myocardial infarction. This policy has been a very important factor in keeping our operative mortality extremely low.

We have been criticized for this throughout the years, particularly by those who have been keen about revascularizing hearts using the aorto-coronary vein bypass grafts. In fact, many have actually proceeded with vein bypass grafts shortly after myocardial infarction had occurred. Recently Dr. Duff's opinion has been confirmed by Dr. Denton Cooley, of the Texas Heart Institute in Houston, who has reported a 14.5 percent operative mortality in patients who underwent aorto-coronary vein bypass grafts when there had been a recent acute myocardial infarction two months or less prior to surgery.

Those performing internal mammary artery implants who ignore this fundamental fact, will have an operative mortality rate higher than 2 percent from the complications of the myocardial infarction alone.

Dr. Duff advised against implantation of internal mammary arteries into hearts of patients with advanced diabetes because in such patients he stated, "The intramyocardial arterioles become atherosclerotic. In such cases branches of the internal mammary artery would join with diseased myocardial arterioles which would be just as unsatisfactory as joining the artery to a diseased surface coronary artery."

Hearts of far advanced hypertensive patients, like those of advanced diabetic cases, have advanced atherosclerosis of their intramyocardial arterioles so that their branching, nondiseased internal mammary arteries connect with atherosclerotic myocardial arterioles.

I won't go into a description of our technique for the preparation of the internal mammary artery prior to its implantation into the human heart. But I will make mention of some of the modifications that have been developed and used by others, such as the use of clamps and silver clips to free the artery from the sternum which damages the artery. In our preparation, the side branches of the internal mammary artery are tied with very fine silk about the thickness of a spider's web, and the artery is gently teased away from the sternum, not removed by the use of scissors or a cautery. We carefully separate the artery from the vein, sternal muscles, and tendons which surround it, so that when it branches within the heart muscle tunnel, these useless structures do not interfere with the branches. Dr. William H. Sewell of Sayre, Pennsylvania, modified the preparation of the artery by using a cautery to free the artery, the vein and some of the chest muscle with its tendons in one mass known as the *Sewell pedicle*.

One of the top surgeons of Houston, Texas, unfortunately decided to make the artery bigger by inserting an artery forceps into its cut open end to stretch it. This of course damaged the lining and wall of the artery so that of 18 patients having left ventricular internal mammary artery implants, all arteries were blocked.

We have known since 1949 that an internal mammary artery must be implanted into an area of myocardial ischemia where there is a demand for it in order to have long term patency and continued functioning of the artery. Because it is not needed, an artery implanted into an area supplied by a normal coronary artery blocks over in a few years. This principle has been confirmed and followed most carefully by Dr. Donald Effler, of the Cleveland Clinic in Cleveland, Ohio, and by Dr. Wilfred Bigelow, of Toronto General Hospital, and by many others who have had great success with internal mammary artery implants.

In our practice, before making the tunnel, we sound the wall of the heart with a needle which detects the resistance offered by scar as compared to the softness of ischemic heart muscle. This ensures that the internal mammary artery is implanted in ventricular muscle, not into scar. Clearly, the artery should not be implanted into an area of previous infarction, because the muscle in such an area turns to scar.

For best results an internal mammary artery should be implanted in a deep tunnel about 2 inches long, not a long superficial tunnel as has been practiced by many surgeons. The tunnel should be made with a blunt artery forceps, spreading heart muscle fibers apart, not with a knife as recommended and practiced by Dr. Sewell. The knife cuts the heart fibers which may result in heart failure. The artery should be implanted with one or two side branches open and bleeding. This allows the blood to flow away through the opened myocardial sinusoidal spaces and thus help to keep the artery patent until its branches join with the myocardial arterioles. We always close the end of the artery. We do not leave it open in the tunnel as recommended by Dr. F. Glenn, of New York City in 1950. Dr. W. Dudley Johnson of Milwaukee, Wisconsin modified the process. Instead of implanting the internal mammary artery into the heart muscle alone, he implanted it with six side branches, which are much smaller than the main artery, into six separate tunnels in the heart and left the internal mammary artery on the surface of the heart. It is my belief that modifications such as these account for the less effective results that some surgeons have reported.

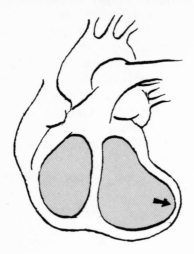 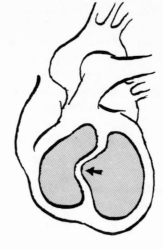

Fig. 25. Aneurysm-septum, left ventricle.   Fig. 26. Aneurysm-external wall,
                                                         left ventricle.

Hope For Those With Blocked Aorto-Coronary Vein Bypass Grafts

In the past few years we have developed techniques to implant an artery or arteries into the hearts of patients whose aorto-coronary vein bypass grafts have blocked. In such cases we have used the internal mammary arteries if they have not been damaged during the aorto-coronary vein bypass operation. If we believe that they have been than we bring an artery which normally supplies the stomach into the chest and implant it into the heart.

We have had great success with this procedure in improving patients still disabled after aorto-coronary vein bypass grafts.

I should mention two other conditions which may develop as a result of myocardial ischemia, caused by obstructed coronary artery atherosclerosis and which may require surgery.

The first is the repair of a blowout area in the wall of the heart. When an area of the heart muscle receives insufficient blood supply, it dies and the patient has a heart attack. This area is then converted into scar. If it is a large scar, it gradually may be stretched by the pressures within the pumping heart chamber and form what we call a *ventricular aneurysm*. This is the blowout.

The operation is a comparatively simple one, involving cutting away the scar, often 2–3 inches in diameter, and sewing the heart

148

wall back together. When accompanied by some form of revascularization this greatly improves the function of the heart.

The second condition relates to the infarction of papillary muscles which control mitral and tricuspid valves. When they are damaged, the valves leak. Such valves may have to be replaced at the same time as a revascularization operation is carried out. This is comparatively rare.

Heart Transplants

Perhaps here I should make mention of heart transplantation. I remember how excited I was when I heard about the work done by Dr. Christian Barnard. My immediate reaction was to consider it terrific, a great breakthrough. Then I began to think about it. I wondered, for instance, why Dr. Norman Shumway, of San Francisco, who had done extensive experimental work while with Dr. Owen Wangensteen of the University of Minnesota Medical Center, had not carried on with the human heart transplant. I then realized the problem. It was not because of technical difficulties but rather because in the animal, there had been very active rejection of the donor's heart. This was also true in the case of a large series of animals tested by Dr. Adrian Kantrowtiz, of Brooklyn, New York.

I then considered the question of allergies. How successful had our allergists been in preventing the recurrence of hay fever, which is caused by a foreign protein? Some success had been achieved but there were still a great number of hay fever sufferers around. If immunologists were unable to desensitize a human being against a ragweed protein or some other protein, it seemed inconceivable they would be able to desensitize a recipient against the multiple complex proteins present in a donor's heart.

My next thought was that the donor's heart, after being sewn into its new location in the patient, would be subjected to the same factors that had caused the recipient's heart to develop coronary artery atherosclerosis. Thus a young heart placed into an older man's body would be bathed in the same atherosclerotic milieu that had caused the coronary arteries to become diseased in the recipient's heart.

On many occasions I have brought these two major facts forth as objections to the principle of human heart transplantation. Thus, from the beginning I have lectured in favor of early revascularization surgery primarily by myocardial implants and supplementary operations to prevent the necessity of human heart transplants. Today, six years later, I am of the same opinion, with regard to patients with coronary artery disease, particularly since a new procedure known as the aorto-coronary vein bypass graft has been added.

There seems to be evidence that the rejection factor, although not overcome, has been reduced by newer advances in immunology. Dr. Shumway has a most encouraging record of successful heart transplants, particularly in hearts that are failing from primary disease of ventricular muscle—but not from disease of coronary arteries or valves.

Unlike coronary arteries, internal mammary arteries do not develop atherosclerosis. They remain open and functioning many years after the patient's own coronary arteries have become occluded by progressive atherosclerosis. Thus heart transplants for very selected patients holds considerable hope when all else fails.

General Advice

I have tried to describe in simplest terms the various kinds of operations available to those in need of heart surgery. But a few words of general advice might be appropriate at this point.

See your family doctor regularly. I can't emphasize this too strongly. Don't wait until you're sick to get a checkup.

If you have pain and your physician says it's anginal and recommends seeing a cardiologist, do so without delay.

See your cardiologist and accept his treatment for at least one year.

If, at the end of the year, you still have anginal pain with or without shortness of breath and are easily fatigued, you should have a cine coronary angiogram performed to determine whether or not surgery is required.

If your cardiologist is not connected with a center that does this kind of testing, seek out another cardiologist. It is *important* that the condition of your coronary artery pipelines be known.

In looking for a cardiologist, try to find one who works closely with a surgeon—and, of course, try to locate one close to your home.

Inquire about the center you pick. Select one where the surgeons and cardiologists work together and where there are at least ten heart operations performed per week.

Pick a center experienced in heart operations. There are many medical centers in Canada and the United States where you can be assured of good attention and good surgery.

CHAPTER 10

Your Heart and the Family Tree

The man sits nervously across the desk from me, folding and unfolding his hands and stammering through his sentences. His brother has developed a heart condition and he is afraid he may be next in line.

"My father died of coronary artery heart disease and so did *his* father before him," he says. "Is it possible that it runs in the family?"

I don't know how many times I've been asked that question over the years. Hundreds of times probably.

"Yes, it's possible to inherit tendencies for certain heart conditions," I tell the man.

It's a mistake to make light of questions such as this. There is just too much evidence to support the existence of hereditary factors in heart disease. Someone once noted facetiously, "If you want to avoid coronary artery heart disease, pick your ancestors."

While there is more truth than humor to the remark, it is dangerous to encourage an individual in the belief that hereditary patterns must determine his health and well-being.

Change your heredity? Pick your ancestors? No, you can't do

that. But the knowledge that a certain disease is prevalent in a family tree should be a warning—and forewarned is forearmed.

"We're a family of heavy people," a fat patient of mine once complained. "My parents are overweight and so are my grandparents. I guess I just come by it naturally."

"I don't buy that philosophy," I answered. "Unless there is glandular trouble (which is rare among males) there is nothing natural about a person being fat. In most cases, he is fat because he eats the wrong things and too much of them, and because he exercises too little."

Families share not only genes but also a great variety of living habits. It is no myth that the child learns from its parents and that it is in childhood that the patterns of life begin to form. A boy learns how to use tools from his father, a girl adopts her mother's methods of cooking—and both grow up practicing the eating habits they developed in the home.

In a very real sense, prevention of coronary artery heart disease begins right there—in the home. We are wiser now than we once were and some of the rules of good health are changing. We know that an infant needs good, wholesome nutrition to grow up strong and healthy but we are also aware of the dangers of overfeeding. Today's roly-poly baby could be tomorrow's obese adult.

The onus here is clearly on the parents. The work of prevention should be in full swing in the formative years, particularly in the case of families with a history of heart disease. Permissive parents are responsible for many of the ills that befall their children in later life—and food is one of the real danger areas.

Don't praise children for eating everything in sight.

Don't encourage second helpings.

Don't let the preschoolers fill up on candy and soft drinks.

Don't let the teenagers fill up on french fries and milkshakes.

Use vegetable or corn oil margarine. Don't buy butter.

Start the children on skim milk right away. Don't have high-cholesterol whole milk in the house.

Prepare the new low-calorie, low-cholesterol desserts. Have ice milk instead of ice cream. If possible, have ice skim milk instead of ice milk.

Above all, strongly discourage smoking.

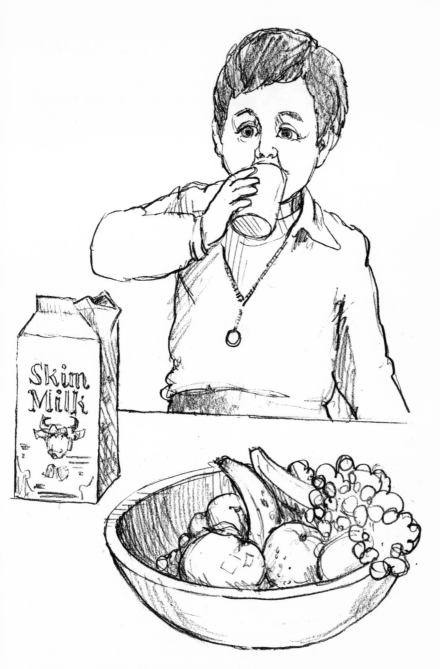

Good eating habits should start early.

Just as training for good eating habits should start early, so should training for exercise. We tend to think that youngsters get all the physical activity they require just by running about. But in a great many cases, this is just not so. Mechanization has virtually eliminated most of the chores children of earlier times were expected to do, and the advent of school-bussing has even made walking obsolete.

Our highly motorized age has produced an army of youngsters who won't walk if they can ride. They have to be *trained* in early life. They have to be *taught* the value of proper exercise.

Wise parents can do much to prevent obesity and future heart trouble in their children through food and exercise habits. But their work doesn't end there. They must help their children develop living patterns that will avoid excessive stress. Keeping physically fit is a good way of avoiding stress, but there are psychological aspects of stress, too. Try not to give your children a psychosis about life. For example, don't expect them to crowd too much into a particular time period.

Tell them that life will make certain demands. Tell them there are certain things they will have to do, even if they don't like them. But show them that it is usually possible to cope with one's problems and take them in stride.

Hypertensive people, for example, should be alert to the danger to their children. There is a tendency for hypertension to run in families, so the offspring of an affected family should be tested every six months—certainly every year—for changes in blood pressure.

A similar danger exists in the case of diabetes, another disease that tends to run in families. It is a wise parent who has his children's blood sugars checked at regular intervals.

We don't have all the answers to the question of hereditary illnesses. But we do know, for example, that sudden death may occur repeatedly in successive generations of families as a consequence of hypertension, coronary artery disease, or both. We know that hypertension is three times as frequent among children of hypertensive individuals as among those of normotensive individuals. Similarly, we know that children of obese parents have four times as much obesity as those of nonobese parents, and that diabetes is eight times as common among siblings of diabetic persons as among those of nondiabetic persons.

Hypertension, obesity, and diabetes are all related to coronary artery disease but there are separate statistics for the disease itself. They show that coronary artery ailments are nearly four times as prevalent among children of affected individuals as among those of unaffected parents.

If we accept the theory of heredity, how does a person with a family history of coronary artery disease, or with a history of one of the factors contributing to it, go about coping with the situation?

To begin with, it does not necessarily follow that parents with coronary artery heart disease must produce similarly afflicted children. What must be recognized is the fact that children *may* inherit the illness tendencies of their elders.

The individual must stick to logic and not let his fears run away with him. I have been preaching this philosophy all my life. There is no need to be afraid if you understand your heart. And that was my reason for writing this book—to help families to live a healthier, happier life with their hearts.

APPENDIX A

Resuscitation

Many a victim of coronary artery heart disease has died of a sudden heart arrest simply because no one who was with him at the time of the attack was familiar with the art of resuscitation. It is sad indeed to hear of these cases because the simple principle of this emergency measure can be carried out by anyone who takes the trouble to read this, or who joins a Canadian or American Red Cross cardiac resuscitation class to learn the technique of cardiac resuscitation. Relatives of cardiac cases should particularly attend such classes. This should include not only the patient's wife but his older children. This type of approach makes the family aware of the possibility of cardiac arrest. It also makes the child of a patient, suffering from coronary artery disease, more likely to follow the preventive measures which are so essential.

The key word is speed. Resuscitation must be started within three and a half to four minutes (sooner if possible) because the brain dies very quickly without oxygenated blood.

As soon as a case of cardiac arrest occurs, feel for carotid pulse in the neck. If there is none, emergency procedures should go into effect. Have someone call the police and ambulance and commence resuscitation immediately.

Principles of resuscitation for cardiac arrest are (1) speed, (2) patient on back on hard flat surface, (3) open airway, (4) pulmonary ventilation, and (5) extra cardiac compression.

Resuscitation is a two-pronged procedure which includes mouth-to-mouth expired air ventilation and external (manual) heart compression to create artificial circulation. There have been cases of a lone woman performing both procedures, but it is more easily handled by two people. If two persons are on hand, it is then possible to do mouth-to-mouth ventilation and external heart compression at the same time. If only one person is present, however, then the resuscitator should breathe rapidly into the lungs three to five times by the expired air technique which I shall describe, and then start manual heart compression.

Resuscitation: Mouth-to-Mouth

Here are the six steps to successful mouth-to-mouth resuscitation:

1. Place the patient on his back on the floor.
2. Pinch nostrils closed with one hand and place other hand under patient's neck.
3. Lift the neck, allowing the head to tilt back as far as it will go. (The mouth will usually open following this maneuver.)
4. Open your mouth wide, take a deep breath and make an airtight seal over the victim's mouth with your lips.
5. Blow air in forcefully until the patient's chest expands.
6. Repeat the procedure every five seconds.

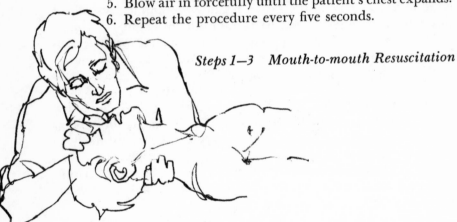

Steps 1—3   Mouth-to-mouth Resuscitation

Steps 4—6   Mouth-to-mouth Resuscitation

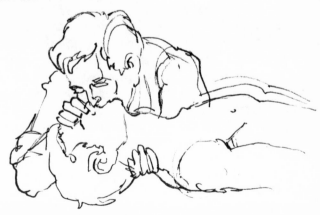

Resuscitation: External Compression

The principle of creating artificial circulation by external heart compression relies upon the fact that the heart occupies most of the space between the breastplate and the spine. Blood is thereby forced out into the body, and most important, to the brain and heart itself. With relaxation, the normal elasticity of the chest wall causes it to spring outward and during this period the heart again fills with blood.

Here are the seven steps to external (manual) heart compression:

1. Place the patient on his back on the floor.
2. Locate the pressure point. This is found on the lower half of the breastplate, just above its soft lower end where it joins the abdomen.
3. Take a position on the left side of the victim. Do not straddle him.
4. Apply both hands to the pressure point parallel with the sternum.

(continues on next page.)

Steps 1—7   Resuscitation: External Compression

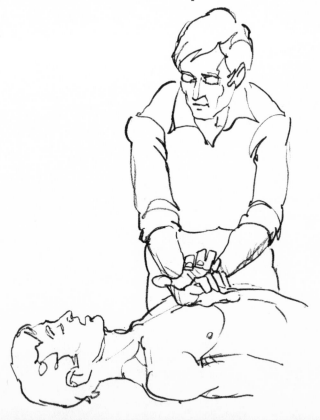

5. Apply firm, heavy pressure through the heel of the hand in contact with the breastplate. Do not apply pressure through the fingers. Push the breastplate in toward the spine about $1\frac{1}{2}$–2 inches.
6. Hold breastplate inward one-half second and then release rapidly.
7. Reapply pressure every second, or at an even faster rate. (A rate of compression slower than 60 times a minute is not beneficial.)

Artificial Ventilation and Circulation

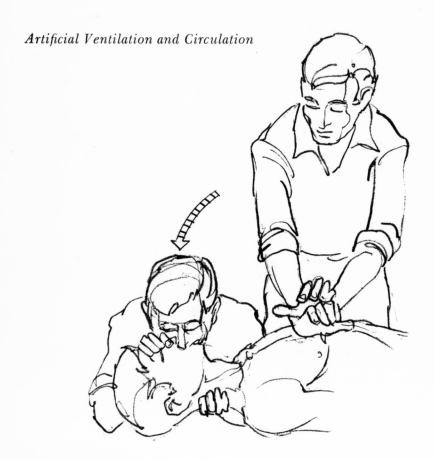

Resuscitation: Artificial Ventilation and Circulation by One Rescuer

Although difficult, one person may provide both adequate artificial ventilation and circulation. When only one person is present when a victim experiences sudden loss of ventilation and heart action, he should first recognize the cardiac arrest and then immediately ventilate the lungs, rapidly, three to five times, by the expired air technique. The rescuer should then very rapidly shift his position slightly and apply manual heart compression 15 times at a rate of once per second. He then quickly shifts again and quickly ventilates two times, immediately returning to heart compression 15 times. He continues this cycle and, as soon as possible, a second person should assume one of his duties. This 15:2 ratio, in spite of its apparent emphasis on circulation, has been demonstrated to provide both adequate ventilation and circulation.

Resuscitation: Artificial Ventilation and Circulation by Two Rescuers

One rescuer immediately ventilates the lungs three to five times by a mouth-to-mouth resuscitation method. The second rescuer immediately provides uninterrupted manual heart compression at a rate to 60 to 80 times a minute while the first rescuer continues mouth-to-mouth resuscitation at the rate of 12 times a minute. Both rescuers continue until the victim begins to breathe normally and heartbeat returns.

How to detect the effectiveness of resuscitation:
1. Pupils previously dilated will constrict.
2. Victim's color will return to normal.
3. Pulse is felt with each artificial compression.
4. Normal respiratory activity may ensue.
5. Normal heart beat is restored.

Warning: Cardiac resuscitation should not be attempted without knowledge of the technique and some practical training. The great single mistake is to press on the upper abdomen instead of the lower chest. This error could result in food and stomach juices coming up into the mouth and entering the lung, thus drowning the victim in his own stomach contents.

APPENDIX B

CHOLESTEROL AND CALORIE DIET CHART

General:

Foods are arranged by category in alphabetical order. Both calorie and cholesterol values are shown. Both usual serving sizes (edible portion) and counts per 100 grams are indicated, these show the relative cholesterol and calorie count of foods.

How to use the chart:

1. See your doctor and show him this diet chart.
2. Total cholesterol intake should be limited to 280 to 300 milligrams (mg.) per day.
3. Total calorie intake should also be limited as follows:

Age in years	Males calorie intake*	Females calorie intake*
6 — 9	2000	2000
9 — 12	2400	2200
12 — 15	2700	2300
15 — 18	3000	2300
18 — 35	2800	2100
35 — 55	2600	1900
55 — 75+	2400	1700

*These figures are based on average height and weight, 5 ft. 4 in. and 128 lbs. for women and 5 ft. 9 in. and 154 lbs. for men.

4. Use diet in conjunction with a realistic exercise programme.

Adhering to these guidelines should assure a balanced and nutritious diet. If you exceed cholesterol count on a given day, try to reduce count on following days to bring the week's average back to the allowable maximum of 300 milligrams of cholesterol per day.

CHOLESTEROL & CALORIE DIET CHART

Food and Description	Household Measure Unit and/or weight	Cholesterol–Calories per Household Measure		Cholesterol–Calories per 100 gm. Portion	
		Cholesterol mg.	Calories approx.	Cholesterol mg.	Calories approx.
BEVERAGES					
Beer	12 oz. (360 gm.)	0	150	0	41
Beef Bouillon Cube	1 cube (4 gm.)	0	5	0	63
Carbonated—Sweetened					
Carbonated Water (Tonic)	10 oz. (305 gm.)	0	95	0	31
Gingerale	10 oz. (305 gm.)	0	95	0	31
Cola	10 oz. (305 gm.)	0	120	0	39
Carbonated Water					
Unsweetened, (Soda)	10 oz. (305 gm.)	0	0	0	0
Chocolate—Drink					
flavored milk with 2% added butter fat	1 c. (250 gm.)	20	190	8	76
chocolate flavored milk	1 c. (250 gm.)	32	212	13	85
hot, homemade	1 c. (250 gm.)	31	238	12	95
cocoa, homemade, with whole milk	1 c. (250 gm.)	35	243	14	97

CHOLESTEROL & CALORIE DIET CHART—Cont'd.

Food and Description	Household Measure Unit and/or weight	Cholesterol–Calories per Household Measure		Cholesterol–Calories per 100 gm. Portion	
		Cholesterol mg.	Calories approx.	Cholesterol mg.	Calories approx.
Low Calorie Beverages	10 oz. (305 gm.)	0	0–10	0	0–3
Milk (see dairy products)					
Spirits—Gin, Rum, Vodka, Whiskey	1½ fluid oz. (42 gm.)	0	105	0	250
Wines					
Dessert Wines	3½ fluid oz. (100 gm.)	0	137	0	137
Dry Table Wine (White, Red)	3½ fluid oz. (100 gm.)	0	85	0	85
BREADS					
White, enriched	1 slice (30 gm.)	trace	82	trace	273
Whole wheat (60%)	1 slice (30 gm.)	trace	72	trace	240
Cornbread					
baked from home recipe made with degermed cornmeal	piece, approx. 2½ x 2½ x 1⅝ in. (83 gm.)	58	172	70	224
baked from mix, made with egg and milk	muffin, approx. 2⅜ in. diam. (40 gm.)	28	93	69	233

baked from mix, made with egg and milk	piece, approx. 2½ x 2½ x 1⅜ in. (55 gm.)	38	128	69	233
Muffins—					
plain, baked from home recipe	muffin, approx. 3 in. diam. (40 gm.)	21	118	53	294

DAIRY PRODUCTS

Butter—					
regular (4 sticks/lb.)	1 tbsp. or ⅛ stick (14 gm.)	35	100	250	714
regular (4 sticks/lb.)	½ c. or 1 stick (113 gm.)	282	810	250	717
whipped (6 sticks or 2, 8 oz. containers/lb.)	1 tbsp. or ⅛ stick (9 gm.)	22	65	250	722
whipped (6 sticks or 2, 8 oz. containers/lb.)	½ c. or 1 stick (76 gm.)	190	540	250	710
Cheese—					
Camembert	1 oz. (28 gm.)	26	84	92	300
Camembert	triangular piece, approx. 2¼ x 2½ x 2½ in., 1⅛ in. high, net wt. 1⅓ oz. (38 gm.)	35	114	92	300
Cheddar, mild or sharp	1 c. shredded (113 gm.)	112	449	99	398
Cheddar, mild or sharp	1 oz. (28 gm.)	28	111	99	398
Colby	1 oz. (28 gm.)	27	111	96	398
Cottage, creamed 1% fat	1 c. packed (267 gm.)	23	183	9	68

165

CHOLESTEROL & CALORIE DIET CHART—Cont'd.

Food and Description	Household Measure Unit and/or weight	Cholesterol–Calories per Household Measure		Cholesterol–Calories per 100 gm. Portion	
		Cholesterol mg.	Calories approx.	Cholesterol mg.	Calories approx.
Cheese cont'd.					
Cottage, creamed 4% fat	1 c. packed (245 gm.)	48	260	19	106
Cottage, uncreamed	1 c. packed (200 gm.)	13	172	7	86
Cream	1 tbsp. (14 gm.)	16	52	114	371
Cream	package, approx. $2\frac{7}{8}$ x 2 x $\frac{7}{8}$ in., net wt. 3 oz. (85 gm.)	94	317	110	373
Edam	1 oz. (28 gm.)	29	87	102	311
Limburger	1 oz. (28 gm.)	28	97	98	345
Mozarrella	1 oz. (28 gm.)	27	96	97	344
Mozarrella, part skim, low moisture	1 oz. (28 gm.)	18	78	66	278
Muenster	1 oz. (28 gm.)	25	105	91	375
Natural, blue	1 oz. (28 gm.)	24	103	87	368
Natural, blue	1 c. crumbled (not packed) (135 gm.)	117	497	86	368
Natural, brick	1 oz. (28 gm.)	25	104	90	370
Neufachatel	package, approx. $2\frac{7}{8}$ x 2 x $\frac{7}{8}$ in., net wt. 3 oz. (85 gm.)	64	277	76	326

Food	Measure				
Pasteurized process cheese—American	slice approx. $3\frac{1}{2}$ x $3\frac{3}{8}$ x $\frac{1}{8}$ in., wt. 1 oz. (28 gm.)	25	104	90	370
Pasteurized process cheese—American spread	1 tbsp. (14 gm.)	9	41	64	288
Pasteurized process cheese—American spread	slice, approx. $2\frac{3}{4}$ x $2\frac{1}{4}$ x $\frac{1}{4}$ in. wt. 1 oz. (28 gm.)	18	81	64	289
Pasteurized process cheese—American spread	1 c. shredded (packed) (113 gm.)	73	327	64	289
Pasteurized process cheese—American food	1 tbsp. (14 gm.)	10	46	72	323
Pasteurized process cheese—American food	slice, approx. $3\frac{1}{2}$ x $3\frac{3}{8}$ x $\frac{1}{8}$ in., wt. 1 oz. (28 gm.)	20	91	71	325
Parmesan	1 oz. (28 gm.)	27	110	95	393
Provolne	1 oz. (28 gm.)	28	98	101	349
Ricotta	1 oz. (28 gm.)	14	46	51	166
Ricotta, part skim	1 oz. (28 gm.)	9	36	32	130
Straws	10 pieces, each 5 in. long, $\frac{3}{8}$ in. wide, $\frac{3}{8}$ in. high (60 gm.)	19	272	32	453
Swiss American	slice, approx. $3\frac{1}{2}$ x $3\frac{3}{8}$ x $\frac{1}{8}$ in., wt. 1 oz. (28 gm.)	26	99	93	355
Swiss	slice, rectangular, approx. $7\frac{1}{2}$ to $7\frac{3}{4}$ x 4 x 1/16 in., wt. $1\frac{1}{4}$ oz. (35 gm.)	35	130	100	371
Welsh rarebit	1 c. (232 gm.)	71	415	31	179

CHOLESTEROL & CALORIE DIET CHART—Cont'd.

Food and Description	Household Measure	Cholesterol—Calories per Household Measure		Cholesterol—Calories per 100 gm. Portion	
	Unit and/or weight	Cholesterol mg.	Calories approx.	Cholesterol mg.	Calories approx.
Cream—					
heavy whipping (unwhipped) (35% fat)	1 tbsp. (15 gm.)	20	53	133	352
half and half (cream and milk)	1 tbsp. (15 gm.)	6	20	42	133
light, coffee or table cream (18% fat)	1 tbsp. (15 gm.)	10	32	66	213
sour cream (10%–18% fat)	1 tbsp. (12 gm.)	8	23	66	192
Ice Cream—					
frozen custard or French ice cream	1 c. (133 gm.)	97	323	73	243
rich, approx. 16% fat	1 c. (148 gm.)	85	329	57	222
regular, approx. 10% fat	1 c. (133 gm.)	53	257	40	193
Ice Milk—					
soft serve	1 c. (175 gm.)	36	265	20	151
hardened	1 c. (131 gm.)	26	200	20	152

Eggs—					
cheese souffle, from home recipe	portion, ¼ of 7-in. diam. souffle (110 gm.)	184	240	167	218
chicken eggs—raw or cooked with nothing added (refuse: shell, 11%)	large egg (50 gm.)	252	82	504	163
scrambled or omelet with milk and fat	omelet, prepared using 1 large egg (64 gm.)	263	111	411	173
Egg substitute	¼ c. (60 gm.)	2	90	3	150
Yolks—raw or cooked with nothing added	yolk from large egg (179 gm.)	252	623	1480	348
Milk—					
buttermilk, fluid, cultured, made from nonfat fluid milk	1 c. (245 gm.)	5	88	0	36
condensed, sweetened	1 c. (306 gm.)	105	982	34	321
dry whole, instant	1¾ c. (120 gm.)	131	602	109	502
evaporated, unsweetened	1 c. (252 gm.)	79	345	31	137
Nonfat, instant, dry	1⅓ c. low density or high density (91 gm.)	20	327	22	359

CHOLESTEROL & CALORIE DIET CHART—Cont'd.

Food and Description	Household Measure Unit and/or weight	Cholesterol—Calories per Household Measure		Cholesterol—Calories per 100 gm. Portion	
		Cholesterol mg.	Calories approx.	Cholesterol mg.	Calories approx.
Milk cont'd.					
Skim milk (nonfat)	1 c. (245 gm.)	5	88	2	36
Whole (3.5% fat)	1 c. (244 gm.)	34	161	14	66
1% fat with 1 to 2% nonfat milk	1 c. (246 gm.)	14	103	6	41
2% fat with 1 to 2% nonfat milk	1 c. (246 gm.)	22	145	9	58
Yoghurt—made from fluid and dry nonfat milk:					
fruit flavored (all kinds)	carton: net wt. 8 oz. (227 gm.)	15	245	7	106
plain	carton: net wt. 8 oz. (227 gm.)	17	125	8	55
vanilla	carton: net wt. 8 oz. (227 gm.)	17	195	8	86

*FATS

	1 c. (205 gm.)				
lard	1 c. (205 gm.)	195	95	1849	902
Margarine—					
All vegetable fat—regular	1 tbsp. or ⅛ stick (14 gm.)	0	0	100	714
⅔ animal fat, ⅓ vegetable fat	1 tbsp. or ⅛ stick (14 gm.)	7	50	100	714
Oils:					
Saturated Oils					
Coconut Oil	1 tbsp. (14 gm.)	0	0	125	893
Monounsaturated Oils					
Olive Oil	1 tbsp. (14 gm.)	0	0	125	893
Peanut Oil	1 tbsp. (14 gm.)	0	0	125	893
Polyunsaturated Oils					
Corn Oil	1 tbsp. (14 gm.)	0	0	125	893
Cottonseed Oil	1 tbsp. (14 gm.)	0	0	125	893
Safflower Oil	1 tbsp. (14 gm.)	0	0	125	893
Soybean Oil	1 tbsp. (14 gm.)	0	0	125	893
Sunflower Oil	1 tbsp. (14 gm.)	0	0	125	893

*Fats—According to the American Heart Association, 35% of total daily calorie intake should be fat. Of this, 10% should be saturated fatty acids, 10% polyunsaturated fatty acids, 15% monounsaturated fatty acids. See further note in dictionary under Fats and Oils.

CHOLESTEROL & CALORIE DIET CHART—Cont'd.

Food and Description	Household Measure Unit and/or weight	Cholesterol—Calories per Household Measure Cholesterol mg.	Calories approx.	Cholesterol—Calories per 100 gm. Portion Cholesterol mg.	Calories approx.
MEATS					
Beef—composite of retail cuts:					
beef and vegetable stew (canned)	1 c. (245 gm.)	36	194	14	79
beef and vegetable stew cooked (home recipe with lean beef chuck)	1 c. (245 gm.)	63	218	26	89
beef, dried, chipped, creamed	1 c. (245 gm.)	65	377	27	154
beef, cooked, bone removed—lean	piece, approx. $4\frac{1}{8}$ in. long, $2\frac{1}{4}$ in. wide, $\frac{1}{2}$ in. thick, or patty approx. 3 in. diam., $\frac{5}{8}$ in. thick, wt. 3 oz. (85 gm.)	80	185	94	217
lean, trimmed of separable fat—cooked	piece or patty approx. $4\frac{1}{8}$ in. long, $2\frac{1}{4}$ in. wide, $\frac{1}{2}$ in. thick or patty approx. 3 in. diam., $\frac{5}{8}$ in. thick, wt. 3 oz. (85 gm.)	77	189	91	220

heart cooked, lean	1 c. chopped or diced pieces (145 gm.)	398	272	274	187
beef, potpie, commercial, frozen, unheated	pie (216 gm.)	38	415	18	192
potpie, home prepared, baked	piece, ⅓ of 9-in. diam. pie (210 gm.)	44	519	21	246
Kidney—all kinds (beef, calf, hog, lamb, cooked)	1 c. sliced pieces, approx. ¼ in. thick (140 gm.)	1125	352	804	252
Lamb—composite of retail cuts:					
cooked, bone removed	2 pieces, approx. 4⅛ in. long, 2¼ in. wide, ¼ in. thick: wt. 3 oz. (85 gm.)	83	235	98	276
lean, trimmed of separable fat, cooked	2 pieces, approx. 4⅛ in. long, 2¼ in. wide, ¼ in. thick: wt. 3 oz. (85 gm.)	85	155	100	182
with bone (refuse bone 16%)	chop, broiled; wt. 4 oz. (112 gm.)	79	400	71	357
without bone, lean only	chop, broiled; wt. 2.6 oz. (74 gm.)	52	140	71	189

173

CHOLESTEROL & CALORIE DIET CHART—Cont'd.

Food and Description	Household Measure / Unit and/or weight	Cholesterol–Calories per Household Measure		Cholesterol–Calories per 100 gm. Portion	
		Cholesterol mg.	Calories approx.	Cholesterol mg.	Calories approx.
Liver— chicken, cooked	liver, approx. 2 in. long, 2 in. wide, $\frac{5}{8}$ in. thick (25 gm.)	187	41	746	165
including beef, calf, hog and lamb, cooked	slice, approx. $6\frac{1}{2}$ in. long, $2\frac{3}{8}$ in. wide, $\frac{3}{8}$ in. thick: wt. 3 oz. (85 gm.)	372	210	438	248
turkey, all classes, cooked	1 c. chopped (140 gm.)	839	246	599	174
Rabbit— domesticated, flesh only, cooked, stewed	1 c. chopped or diced (140 gm.)	127	302	91	216

Pork—					
cooked—composite of all cuts, lean, trimmed of separable fats	2 pieces, approx. 4⅛ in. long, 2¼ in. wide, ¼ in. thick: wt. 3 oz. (85 gm.)	75	209	88	247
bone removed, cooked	2 pieces, approx. 4⅛ in. long, 2¼ in, wide, ¼ in. thick: wt. 3 oz. (85 gm.)	76	310	89	364
Sausage—					
frankfurter, cooked, all meat	1 frank, 8/lb. (56 gm.)	34	170	62	304
Sweetbreads (thymus)—					
cooked	3 oz. (85 gm.)	386	188	466	221
*Veal—*composite of retail cuts:					
cooked, bone removed	piece, approx. 2½ in. long, 2½ in. wide, ⅜ in. thick: wt. 3 oz. (85 gm.)	86	185	101	217
lean, trimmed of separable fat, cooked	piece, approx. 2½ in. long, 2½ in. wide, ⅜ in. thick: wt. 3 oz. (85 gm.)	84	185	99	217

CHOLESTEROL & CALORIE DIET CHART—Cont'd.

Food and Description	Household Measure Unit and/or weight	Cholesterol—Calories per Household Measure		Cholesterol—Calories per 100 gm. Portion	
		Cholesterol mg.	Calories approx.	Cholesterol mg.	Calories approx.
	PASTA				
macaroni and cheese, baked, made from home recipe	1 c. (200 gm.)	42	430	21	215
spaghetti with meat balls in tomato sauce—canned	1 c. (250 gm.)	39	258	9	103
spaghetti with meat balls in tomato sauce, cooked from home recipe	1 c. (248 gm.)	75	332	30	134
Noodles—					
Whole egg dry form	package, net wt. 8 oz. (227 gm.)	213	883	94	389
whole egg, cooked	1 c. (160 gm.)	50	200	31	125
chow mein noodles—canned	1 c. (45 gm.)	5	220	12	489

PASTRY

Cakes:

angel food, made with water and flavorings, baked from mix	piece, $\frac{1}{2}$ of 10-in. diam. cake (53 gm.)	0	137	0	258
chocolate (devil's food) 2 layer made with eggs, water, chocolate frosting, baked from mix	cupcake, small 2$\frac{1}{2}$ in. diam. (36 gm.)	17	122	47	339
chocolate (devil's food) 2 layer made with eggs, water, chocolate frosting, baked from mix	piece 1/16 of 9-in. diam. cake (69 gm.)	33	234	48	339
chocolate (devil's food) 2 layer with chocolate frosting baked from home recipe	piece 1/16 of 9-in. diam. cake (75 gm.)	32	277	43	369
fruitcake, dark, home recipe	slice, 1/30 of 8-in. loaf (15 gm.)	7	57	45	380
gingerbread, made with water, mix	piece 1/9 of 8-in. sq. cake (63 gm.)	trace	174	1	276
popovers, baked from home recipe	1 popover, approx. 2$\frac{3}{4}$ in. diam. at top (yield from $\frac{1}{4}$ c. batter) (40 gm.)	59	90	147	224

CHOLESTEROL & CALORIE DIET CHART—Cont'd.

Food and Description	Household Measure Unit and/or weight	Cholesterol–Calories per Household Measure		Cholesterol–Calories per 100 gm. Portion	
		Cholesterol mg.	Calories approx.	Cholesterol mg.	Calories approx.
Cakes cont'd.					
sponge cake—home recipe	piece 1/12 of 10-in. diam. cake (66 gm.)	162	196	246	297
white, 2 layer made with egg whites, chocolate frosting, baked from mix	piece 1/16 of 9-in. diam. cake (71 gm.)	1	249	2	351
yellow, 2 layer with chocolate frosting—home recipe	piece, 1/16 of 9-in. diam. cake (75 gm.)	33	274	44	365
yellow, 2 layer, made with egg, water, chocolate frosting, baked from mix	piece, 1/16 of 9-in. diam. cake (75 gm.)	36	253	48	337
cream puffs with custard filling	1 cream puff, approx. 3½ in. diam., 2 in. high (130 gm.)	188	303	144	233
Cookies:					
brownies with nuts, baked from home recipe	1 brownie, approx. 1¾ x 1¾ x ⅞ in. (20 gm.)	17	97	83	485
lady fingers	4 ladyfingers, approx. 3¼ x 1⅜ x 1⅛ in. (44 gm.)	157	158	356	360

Pancakes— baked from mix, made with egg and milk	$\frac{1}{2}$ in. thick (yield from approx. 7 tbsp. batter) (73 gm.)	54	164	74	225
Pies:					
custard, baked	sector $\frac{1}{8}$ of 9-in. diam. pie (114 gm.)	120	249	105	218
lemon meringue	sector $\frac{1}{8}$ of 9-in. diam. pie (105 gm.)	98	268	93	255
lemon chiffon	sector $\frac{1}{8}$ of 9-in. diam. pie (81 gm.)	137	254	169	314
pumpkin, baked	sector $\frac{1}{8}$ of 9-in. diam. pie (232 gm.)	70	490	61	211
Waffles— baked from mix, made with egg and milk	1 waffle, 9 x 9 x $\frac{5}{8}$ in. (yield from approx. 1$\frac{1}{8}$ c. batter) (200 gm.)	119	505	60	275

POULTRY

Chicken—all classes					
breasts, cooked total edible	meat and skin from $\frac{1}{2}$ breast (from 3 lb. ready-to-cook chicken, raw) (92 gm.)	74	151	80	164
breasts, meat only	meat from $\frac{1}{2}$ breast (from 3 lb. ready-to-cook chicken, raw) (80 gm.)	63	163	79	203

CHOLESTEROL & CALORIE DIET CHART—Cont'd.

Food and Description	Household Measure Unit and/or weight	Cholesterol–Calories per Household Measure Cholesterol mg.	Calories approx.	Cholesterol–Calories per 100 gm. Portion Cholesterol mg.	Calories approx.
Chicken cont'd.					
drumstick, cooked, total edible	meat and skin from 1 drumstick (from 3 lb. ready-to-cook chicken, raw) (52 gm.)	47	79	91	151
drumstick, meat only	meat and skin from 1 drumstick (from 3 lb. ready-to-cook chicken, raw) (43 gm.)	39	101	91	234
flesh and skin only, cooked	flesh and skin from 3 lb. ready-to-cook chicken, raw (624 gm.)	542	1560	87	250
chicken à la king, cooked from home recipe	1 c. (245 gm.)	185	468	76	191
chicken and noodles	1 c. (240 gm.)	96	367	40	153
fricasse, cooked from home recipe	1 c. (240 gm.)	96	386	40	161
potpie, commercial, frozen, unheated	pie (227 gm.)	29	497	13	219

180

	1	2	3	4
potpie, home prepared, baked	piece $\frac{1}{3}$ of 9-in. diam. pie (232 gm.)	71	545	31	235
heart, chicken, cooked all classes	1 c. chopped or diced pieces (145 gm.)	335	251	231	173
Gizzard:					
chicken, all classes, cooked	yield from 1 lb. raw approx. 12$\frac{1}{2}$ oz. (354 gm.)	690	524	195	148
turkey, all classes, cooked	yield from 1 lb. raw approx. 12$\frac{3}{4}$ oz. (361 gm.)	827	708	229	196
Turkey—all classes:					
dark meat without skin, cooked	4 pieces approx. 2$\frac{1}{2}$ in. long, 1$\frac{5}{8}$ in. wide, $\frac{1}{4}$ in. thick: wt. 3 oz. (85 gm.)	86	172	101	203
flesh, skin and giblets, cooked	flesh and skin and giblets from 13$\frac{1}{2}$ lb. ready-to-cook turkey, raw (3,680 gm.)	3864	8390	105	228
flesh and skin only, cooked	flesh and skin from 13$\frac{1}{2}$ lb. ready-to-cook turkey, raw (3,530 gm.)	3283	7871	93	223
light meat, without skin, cooked	2 pieces, approx. 4 in. long, 2 in. wide, $\frac{1}{4}$ in. thick: wt. 3 oz. (85 gm.)	65	149	77	176

181

CHOLESTEROL & CALORIE DIET CHART—Cont'd.

Food and Description	Household Measure	Cholesterol–Calories per Household Measure		Cholesterol–Calories per 100 gm. Portion	
	Unit and/or weight	Cholesterol mg.	Calories approx.	Cholesterol mg.	Calories approx.
Turkey—all classes: cont'd.					
heart, cooked	1 c. chopped or diced pieces (145 gm.)	345	313	238	216
potpie, commercial, frozen, unheated	pie, net wt. 8 oz. (227 gm.)	20	447	9	197
potpie, home prepared, baked	piece, $\frac{1}{3}$ of 9-in. diam. pie (232 gm.)	71	550	31	237
PUDDINGS					
bread with raisins	1 c. (265 gm.)	170	504	64	190
chocolate, made from mix, cooked	1 c. (260 gm.)	30	322	12	124

corn	1 c. (245 gm.)	102	255	42	104
custard, baked	1 c. (265 gm.)	278	305	105	115
rice with raisins	1 c. (265 gm.)	29	387	11	146
tapioca cream	1 c. (165 gm.)	159	221	97	134
vanilla (blanc mange) from home recipe	1 c. (255 gm.)	35	283	14	111

SALAD DRESSINGS

cooked, made from home recipe	1 c. (255 gm.)	190	418	74	164
cooked, made from home recipe	1 tbsp. (16 gm.)	12	26	74	164
mayonnaise, commercial	1 c. (220 gm.)	154	1580	70	718
mayonnaise, commercial	1 tbsp. (14 gm.)	10	101	70	718
mayonnaise—type commercial	1 c. (235 gm.)	118	1018	50	733
mayonnaise—type commercial	1 tbsp. (15 gm.)	8	65	50	433

CHOLESTEROL & CALORIE DIET CHART—Cont'd.

Food and Description	Household Measure Unit and/or weight	Cholesterol—Calories per Household Measure		Cholesterol—Calories per 100 gm. Portion	
		Cholesterol mg.	Calories approx.	Cholesterol mg.	Calories approx.
SAUCES					
cheese	1 c. (250 gm.)	44	433	18	173
tartar, regular	1 c. (230 gm.)	118	1221	837	531
tartar, regular	1 tbsp. (14 gm.)	7	74	51	531
white, thick	1 c. (250 gm.)	30	495	12	198
white, medium	1 c. (250 gm.)	33	404	13	162
white, thin	1 c. (250 gm.)	36	306	14	122
SEAFOOD & FISH					
Caviar— sturgeon, granular	1 tbsp. (16 gm.)	48	42	300	263
Clams— canned, drained solids	½ c. (80 gm.)	50	78	63	98
hard or round (refuse: shell and liquid 83%)	1 doz. chowder clam; 5 lb. ⅔ oz. yielding approx. 13.7 oz. raw meat (389 gm.)	194	190	50	49

meat only	1 c. (19 large soft clams or 7 round chowders) (227 gm.)	114	90	50	80
soft (refuse: shell and liquid 65%)	1 doz. large clams 14.4 oz. yielding approx. 5 oz. raw meat (143 gm.)	72	117	50	82
fritters	1 fritter (2 in. diam. 1¾ in. thick) (40 gm.)	51	124	129	311
Crab—all kinds					
crab, imperial, all kinds	1 c. (220 gm.)	308	323	140	147
deviled, all kinds	1 c. (210 gm.)	244	395	102	188
meat only, canned, all kinds	1 c. packed (160 gm.)	161	162	101	101
steamed in shell (refuse: shell 52%) meat only	1 c. (125 gm.)	125	116	100	93
Cod—					
raw dried, salted	piece approx. 5½ in. long, 1½ in. wide, ½ in. thick (80 gm.)	66	104	82	130
Haddock—					
flesh only, cooked	net wt. 3 oz. (85 gm.)	51	140	60	164
Halibut—					
flesh only, cooked, broiled with vegetable shortening	fillet, approx. 6½ in. long, 2½ in. wide, ⅝ in. thick (125 gm.)	75	214	60	171

CHOLESTEROL & CALORIE DIET CHART—Cont'd.

Food and Description	Household Measure Unit and/or weight	Cholesterol—Calories per Household Measure Cholesterol mg.	Calories approx.	Cholesterol—Calories per 100 gm. Portion Cholesterol mg.	Calories approx.
Herring— canned, plain, solids and liquids	can, size 300 x 407 (no. 300) net wt. 15 oz. (425 gm.)	412	884	97	208
Lobster: meat only, cooked	1 c. cut in ½-in. cubes (145 gm.)	123	137	85	95
Newburg	1 c. (250 gm.)	456	485	182	194
Mackerel— cooked, flesh only, broiled with vegetable shortening	fillet, approx. 8½ in. long, 2½ in. wide, ½ in. thick (105 gm.)	106	247	101	236
flesh only (canned solids and liquids)	can size 300 x 407 (no. 300) net wt. 15 oz. (425 gm.)	399	765	94	180
Oysters— canned, solids and liquids meat only, Eastern and Pacific—raw	3 oz. (85 gm.)	38	65	45	76
	1 c. approx. 13–19 Eastern Selects (medium) 19–31 Eastern standards small, 4–6 Pacific medium or 6–9 Pacific small (240 gm.)	120	158	50	66

raw in shell (Eastern select) (medium size) (refuse: shell and liquor 90%)	12 oysters, about 4 lb. yielding about $6\frac{1}{3}$ oz. meat (180 gm.)	90	119	50	66
Oyster stew, home prepared 1 part oysters to 3 parts whole milk by volume	1 c. (240 gm.)	57	206	24	86
Oyster stew, home prepared, 1 part oysters to 2 parts whole milk by volume	1 c. (240 gm.)	63	233	26	97
Salmon—					
roe, salmon, raw	1 oz. (28 gm.)	101	58	360	207
sockeye or red, canned, solids and liquids	can size 301 x 411 (no. 1 Tall) net wt. 16 oz. (454 gm.)	159	531	35	171
steak, broiled with vegetable shortening (refuse: bone 12%)	piece, approx. $6\frac{3}{4}$ in. long, $2\frac{1}{2}$ in. wide, 1 in. thick (145 gm.)	59	263	47	182
Sardines—					
canned in oil, solids and liquid	can size 405 x 301 x 014 (no. $\frac{1}{4}$ oil) net wt. $3\frac{3}{4}$ oz. (106 gm.)	127	207	120	196
drained solids	can (no. $\frac{1}{4}$ oil) drained, net wt. $3\frac{1}{4}$ oz. (92 gm.)	129	185	140	203

187

CHOLESTEROL & CALORIE DIET CHART—Cont'd.

Food and Description	Household Measure Unit and/or weight	Cholesterol—Calories per Household Measure mg.	approx.	Cholesterol—Calories per 100 gm. Portion mg.	approx.
Scallops— steamed, muscle only	3 oz. (85 gm.)	45	95	53	112
Shrimp— canned, drained solids	1 c. approx. 22 large or 76 small (128 gm.)	192	147	150	115
Tuna— canned in oil, solids and liquid	can, size 307 x 113 (no. ½) chunk style, net wt. 6½ oz. (184 gm.)	100	1394	55	288
canned in water, solids and liquids	can, size 307 x 113 (no. ½) chunk style, net wt. 6½ oz. (184 gm.)	116	234	63	127
drained solids	can, (no. ½) chunk style, drained wt. 5½ oz. (157 gm.)	102	309	65	197

*VEGETABLES

Chop Suey— with meat, canned	3 oz. (85 gm.)	10	53	12	62
with meat, cooked from home recipe	1 c. (250 gm.)	64	300	26	120

Chow Mein—Chicken					
without noodles, canned	1 c. (250 gm.)	7	95	3	38
without noodles, cooked from home recipe	1 c. (250 gm.)	77	255	31	102
Pepper—sweet—					
stuffed with beef and crumbs	pepper approx. 2¾ in. long, 2½ in. diam. with 1⅛ c. stuffing (185 gm.)	56	315	30	170
Potatoes—					
au gratin, made with milk and cheese	1 c. (245 gm.)	36	355	15	145
potato salad from home recipe made with mayonnaise and hard cooked eggs	1 c. (250 gm.)	162	363	65	145
scalloped, made with milk	1 c. (245 gm.)	14	255	6	104

*Vegetables—All vegetables contain no cholesterol unless prepared with other ingredients. Calorie content varies widely.

APPENDIX C

EXERCISE CHART

General:

This chart is designed to help you prevent coronary heart disease. Proper exercise has been proven to reduce the blood cholesterol levels, besides training the cardiovascular system for endurance by making your system work harder for sustained periods.

How to use the chart:

1. Select your age group and conditioning capabilities from the chart. Be honest with yourself. Your doctor will give you an evaluation if any doubt exists.
2. Decide what kind of exercise within your conditioning capabilities you would like to do on a regular basis. This program offers several choices. A combination of two or more activities are often effective and enjoyable.
3. Perform the exercise or activity on a planned basis, if possible daily, but certainly 3 times a week.
4. Use in conjunction with the Cholesterol and Calorie Diet Chart on page 162.

Note:

Moderate, severe and very severe exercise increases metabolism so that more calories are used during the 24 hours following exercise.

All men over 40 before embarking in a program of conditioning should consult their physician to make certain that their heart, blood vessels, blood pressure and their lungs are functioning normally and to find out how much weight they must lose before starting the program in order to avoid a catastrophe.

TYPES OF EXERCISES RECOMMENDED FOR THOSE WITHOUT CORONARY HEART DISEASE

Type of Exercise	Value of Exercises in training Cardiovascular System for Endurance	Reported Calories Used	Exercises Recommended at Different Ages Providing There Is No Evidence of Heart or Lung Disease				Remarks
			Up to 25	25–40	40–65	65–75	
Calisthenics or setting up exercise yoga	None	about 100/hr.	Yes	Yes	Yes	Yes	These exercises do not stress the cardiovascular system but are valuable in muscle toning and stress reduction
Static or isometric contractions	None	about 100/hr.	Yes	Yes	Yes	Yes	These exercises do not stress the cardiovascular system but are valuable in muscle toning

Type of Exercise	Value of Exercises in training Cardiovascular System for Endurance	Reported Calories Used	Exercises Recommended at Different Ages Providing There Is No Evidence of Heart or Lung Disease				Remarks
			Up to 25	25–40	40–65	65–75	
Light Exercise tennis doubles, squash doubles, handball doubles, slow walking, golf (if person walks), gardening, bicycling	Some Value	170–200/hr.	Yes	Yes	Yes	Yes	Light exercise should be undertaken by all ages to start with if they have not been exercising for some years and should be performed in moderation
Moderate Exercise walking not fast alternating with slow jogging, 5BX plan,	Great Value	300–450/hr.	Yes	Yes	Yes	Yes	Moderate exercise is allowed for those who have no proven cardio-vascular disease and

cross country skiing (moderate), horse-back riding, swimming, down hill skiing, | | | | | | are not overweight and for those who have maintained a program of exercise throughout the years

| *Severe Exercise* very fast walking alternating with slow jogging, handball—singles, tennis—singles, squash—singles, long distance cross country skiing (strenuous), downhill skiing (competitive), martial arts (competitive) | Excellent | 600–650/hr. | Yes | Yes | No* | No | Severe exercise stresses the cardiovascular system. There is an increase in blood pressure and pulmonary pressure except with very fast walking. |

*There are exceptions here, but a doctor's advice and top physical conditioning are mandatory.

Type of Exercise	Value of Exercises in training Cardiovascular System for Endurance	Reported Calories Used	Exercises Recommended at Different Ages Providing There Is No Evidence of Heart or Lung Disease					Remarks
			Up to 25	25–40	40–65	65–75		
*Very Severe*** *Exercise* Mountain climbing, crew racing, hard continuous jogging	Excellent	600/hr.	Yes	Yes	No	No		A high percentage of the total cardiac output is used by the skeletal muscles depriving the kidneys, spleen, stomach of an adequate source of oxygenated blood to an extent that members of crews after a race show albumen cast and blood in their urine

**Should be avoided by all except those in top physical condition.

Sources include Geoffrey H. Bourne, Under Chapter on Nutrition and Exercise. Exercise Physiology by Harold B. Falls Academic Press, New York and London, 1968.

The Heart Dictionary

Adrenal cortex   The outer layer of the adrenal gland which secretes hormones.

Adrenal gland   A gland located near the kidney. It is composed of two major parts—the center part, medulla, secretes epinephrine, the outer part secretes cortisone.

Anger   An emotion which results in raised blood pressure, increased heart rate, and constriction of arteries throughout the body. The elevated blood pressure increases the work of the heart. If some part of the heart muscle has insufficient oxygenated blood (myocardial ischemia) to meet the demand, signals go out to the brain and patient may feel anginal pain.

Angina decubitus   Pain of heart (angina pectoris) occurring while lying down.

Angina pectoris   A condition marked by paroxysmal chest pain with a feeling of suffocation. Often described as having a constricting band around chest or "elephant sitting on chest." Pain may radiate down left or right arms or both; to neck or shoulders or between shoulder blades. It is a red light signal, warning the patient of a lack of oxygenated blood to the heart muscle (myocardium) caused by diseasesd coronary arteries. Brought on by effort or excitement, it may disappear spontaneously, and be relieved by rest or nitroglycerine within a few minutes. Condition was first described by Heberden in 1768.
   See also Persistent anginal pain.

Angina pectoris—pain after eating   Occurs in some, cause unknown. May be confused with pain of abdominal origin.

Anterior descending coronary artery Branch of left coronary artery which descends upon the front of the left ventricular wall. Through its branches it supplies the pumping muscle in the front of the heart, and sometimes part of the back of the left ventricle, with oxygenated blood. It also supplies part of the wall dividing the right and left ventricular chambers known as the inter ventricular septum.

Aorta Largest artery in the body. It leaves the left ventricle to give arterial branches to entire system, including the coronary arteries—its first branches.

Arterial blood (oxygenated) Arterial blood is oxygenated. While going through the lungs the red blood cells and plasma have picked up oxygen, thus making arterial blood bright red.

Arteries *See* Blood vessels.

Arteriole A minute arterial branch, especially one just proximal to a capillary.

Arteriosclerosis A condition marked by loss of elasticity, and by thickening and hardening of the arteries.

Atherosclerosis A condition occurring in large and medium size arteries with deposits in the intima (inner lining of arteries) of yellowish plaques containing lipoid material and cholesterol.

Atria or Auricles Small, thin-walled collecting heart chambers located on top of the right and left ventricles. Right atrium collects venous blood from body. Left atrium collects arterial blood from lungs.

Autopsy The postmortem examination of a body, that is, the examination after death.

Autopsy room A room in which pathologists perform autopsies.

Blockage Any blocking, stoppage, obstruction, or closure.

Blood The fluid pumped by the heart to every cell in the body. It is composed of oxygen-carrying red cells, white cells which fight bacterial invaders and fluid plasma in which red and white cells float. The fluid part of the blood contains nutrient substances such as sugar, proteins, amino acids, salts, fats, lipoproteins (containing cholesterol), hormones, and vitamins. Also contained in the blood are waste products of the body such as carbon dioxide and urea, which are eliminated by the lungs, kidneys, and skin.

Blood clotting time Normal bleeding from a blood vessel is stopped by the clotting of blood. Usual clotting time is 10 minutes. Prolonged clotting time of 18 minutes or longer means greater blood loss during surgery. On the other hand, shortened clotting time may favor clotting inside diseased coronary artery, which could result in blockage and possible myocardial infarction.

Blood pressure Pressure in large

arteries leaving the great aorta when left ventricle contracts and relaxes. There are two arterial pressures: first, systolic, top pressure during left ventricular contraction; and second, diastolic, arterial pressure when left ventricle is resting. Normal systolic pressure for men averages 120 millimeters of mercury; diastolic pressure, about 80 millimeters of mercury. Normal systolic pressure for women averages 113 millimeters of mercury; diastolic pressure, 70 millimeters of mercury. It does not change much after age 20 unless there is disease. Hypertension is when blood pressure is elevated above normal.

Blood vessels   There are three major systems:
1. *Arteries.* The vessels through which oxygenated blood is carried from the heart to every part of the body. The arterial tree begins with the largest artery in the body, the aorta, which leaves the left ventricle, runs through the chest and abdomen. It is the size of a radiator hose in an automobile.

On its way this large arterial pipeline sends out branches to feed all parts of the body. Like a tree, the further away from the trunk, the smaller the branches, eventually reaching the tissues where the small arteries end in the capillary networks.

All arteries are hollow tubes lined with a smooth glistening tissue, the endothelium which is made of flat pavement-like cells.

The endothelium with an outer elastic layer is called the intima. Surrounding the intima is a thick layer of muscle tissue. Atherosclerosis involves primarily the intima of arteries.
2. *Veins.* The veins are hollow tubes lined by a smooth tissue made up of endothelium, pavement-like cells. Vein walls are thin. The coating of large veins is same as that of the arteries, but much thinner. They originate on the other side of the capillary networks, collect unoxygenated (used) blood carrying the by-products of metabolism. Small veins join to form larger ones; finally two large veins reach the right atrium from the upper and lower parts of body, respectively. A third vein carrying used blood from the heart also empties into the right atrium. All veins carry venous unoxygenated blood to the heart, except the pulmonary veins which carry oxygenated blood from the lungs back to the left atrium.
3. *Capillaries.* Small microscopic vessels forming networks in all tissues lying between the arterial and venous systems. They are somewhat larger than a red cell, and are thin-walled, thus permitting oxygen and nutrient substances to diffuse through their walls to reach the living tissues.

Brain   Mass of nerve tissue within the skull.

Bundle of His   Named after its discoverer, Dr. Wilhelm His. A small band of unusual heart muscle fibers, originating in the atrioventricular node. In the right atrium it first passes through atrioventricular junction, then beneath the endocardium of the right ventricle on the membranous part of the interventricular septum. It divides into right and left branches at the upper end of the muscular part of the interventricular septum. These branches descend in the septal wall of right and left ventricles to be distributed to those two chambers. The Bundle of His propagates the atrial contraction rhythm to the ventricles. Its interruption produces heart block.

Calcium deposits in coronary arteries Calcium may be deposited in the intima of coronary arteries which have become inflamed through irritation by cholesterol crystals. The process occurs over a period of years, resulting in eventual hardening of the arteries.

Capillaries *See* Blood vessels.

Cardiac output The amount of blood pumped by the left ventricle into the aorta in one minute. An average person has a cardiac output of 5.6 liters per minute with an average pulse of 66 per minute. Stroke volume is output of left ventricle during one contraction. The stroke volume times number of beats per minute equals cardiac output.

Cardiac profile Outline of patient's characteristics said to predispose him to coronary artery heart disease.

Cardiac surgeon A qualified surgeon who is specially trained to operate upon hearts.

Cardiologist A qualified prac-

titioner who is specially trained in the study and medical treatment of heart disease, but does not perform surgery.

Cholesterol A fatlike pearly substance (amonatomical alcohol $C_{27}H_{45}OH$), which crystalizes in the form of circular crystals. When stored in the intima (lining) of the arteries it begins to irritate, and over a period of time sets up an inflammatory reaction which may damage the arterial lining and lead to narrowing of the artery due to atheroma. Cholesterol is found in all animal fats and oils, brain, whole milk, yolk of eggs, liver, kidneys, adrenal glands, and pancreas (sweet breads). It is not found in most vegetable oils (polyunsaturated oils or fats). When taken with food it combines with bile salts to get through bowel membrane and then combines with protein to form a lipoprotein within the cell. From the cell it circulates through the blood as a lipoprotein. It circulates through the entire body. Every body cell membrane is composed of lipoprotein which contains about 40 percent cholesterol. All body cells except those in the brain can make cholesterol, which occurs in cell membrane. It forms the basis of hormones such as those produced by the adrenal gland, ovary, and testicles.

It is carried to arterial endothelium as a lipoprotein and is dissociated from the protein to appear in the intima as needlelike crystals. These set up irritations within the arterial intima and are said to be a cause of atherosclerosis.

It is excreted from the blood

recombined with bile salts through the liver and the gallbladder. Gall stones are primarily composed of cholesterol. It is also excreted in the stool. Elevated blood cholesterol is said to be a factor in the production of atherosclerosis. (See discussion in Chapter 6 and Appendix B.)

Cholesterol deposits in coronary arteries   Usually in intima of coronary arteries, may cause irritation and inflammation.

Cine coronary arteriography
Using special X ray equipment, the image intensifier and a highly complex scientific camera, a moving picture is taken of the inside of each coronary artery. This is done by threading a small hollow plastic tube into a large artery in the arm or leg. Using a television screen, the tube is directed to the mouth of a coronary artery. A dye, visible on a television screen, is injected into each coronary artery separately; its passage down the coronary arterial trunk and its branches is followed by the image intensifier. A moving picture, which outlines the inside of each coronary artery, is taken at the time of the injection, showing whether its lumen is normal, narrowed, or blocked.

At the same investigation the tube is inserted into the cavity of the left ventricle. Dye is injected which outlines the size of the ventricle, and the thickness of its wall. It shows those parts which are contracting and those not contracting due to ischemia and scar. It also shows bulges (ventricular

aneurysms) and defects in the valves.

Circulation   Movement of blood in a regular or circuitous course throughout the body including the heart.

Collaterals   A word used to describe arterial channels on the heart surface or within its muscular walls. They either join the right coronary arterial system with that of the left, or join the two parts of the left coronary arterial system. In human hearts such collateral arterial channels are present in 7 percent of normal hearts. In some they form naturally in response to ischemia caused by disease of a surface coronary artery. Rarely does a collateral form to bring fresh oxygenated blood from one of the pericardial sac vessels. A collateral arterial vessel may channel sufficient oxygenated blood into the area deprived of oxygenated blood due to blockage of its coronary arteries and thus prevent the muscle in the area from dying (or becoming infarcted).
(See Heart attack.)

Coronary arteries   There are two coronary arteries—right and left—which are the first branches that come off the large aorta as it leaves the left ventricle. They turn back to supply the heart muscle with oxygenated blood and many other nutrients. Without adequate oxygen, heart muscle stops contracting and dies.

Coronary arteriogram   The finished film obtained by cine arteriography.

Coronary artery disease, Epidemic in U.S.A. Within 14 years, every eighth man between 40-44 years of age will have a heart attack; also within 14 years every sixth man between 45-49 years of age will have had an attack; every fifth man between 50-54 years of age will have had one; and every fourth man between 55-60 years of age will have had a heart attack. According to recent Framingham studies, (quoted by Dr. W. P. Castelli on August 29, 1974), by the age of 60, every fifth U.S. male has already had a heart attack.

Coronary care unit A specialized area in a hospital where patients with suspected, or with confirmed myocardial infarction (heart attack), are watched and treated by highly trained nurses and cardiologists.

Cortisone A carbohydrate-regulating hormone from the adrenal gland cortex.

Death When the heart stops pumping and cannot be restarted and when all electrical activity ceases in the brain.

Diabetes mellitus A disorder in which the ability to utilize sugars is diminished or lost due to insufficient insulin production by the pancreas. Patients with diabetes tend to develop atherosclerosis more frequently than nondiabetics.

Diastolic blood pressure Minimum arterial pressure when left ventricle relaxes after contracting. Average—75 millimeters of mercury; normal range—60-90 millimeters of mercury.

Digitalis A cardiotonic heart stimulant made from the dried leaf of the plant *Digitalis purpurea* known as the foxglove.

Digitoxin A cardiotonic glycoside obtained from *Digitalis purpurea* and other species of digitalis, used in treatment of congestive heart failure.

Discs in the neck Protrusion of a disc lying between two cervical vertebrae may press on sensory nerve roots of the left arm and left chest. The pain may resemble angina pectoris and may even be relieved by nitroglycerine.

Diuretic A chemical given to increase urine output to remove fluid from lungs, legs, and abdomen.

Dizziness There are many causes, one of which may be atherosclerosis, which narrows the artery and thus reduces the oxygenated blood flow through major arteries leading to the brain.

Electrocardiogram (ECG) A tracing, recorded on paper, of the electrical current produced by the contraction of the heart. The normal electrocardiogram shows upward and downward deflections, the result of auricular and ventricular activity. Variations from normal are detected by the electrocardiogram.

Elevated blood cholesterol According to present North

American standards, normal blood serum cholesterol levels range from 150 to 300 mg. per 100 cc., although most authorities consider levels to be elevated when over 242 mg. per 100 cc. These standards of normal blood serum cholesterol have to be modified along the lines of the cholesterol levels of Eastern nations which have a low coronary artery incidence. We must aim for blood serum cholesterol levels of 180 mg. per 100 cc., and lower, in order to stem the epidemic of coronary artery atherosclerosis.

Endocrine secretion   Internal glandular secretions of hormones into blood or lymph. These hormones have a specific effect on another organ or tissue. They come from the thyroid, testicles, ovaries, pituitary, etc.

Endothelium   A smooth, glistening thin tissue made up of flat pavement-like cells which, in continuity, line the chambers of the heart, arteries, arterioles, capillaries, and veins of entire body.

Enzymes   An organic compound which can accelerate a chemical action.

Epicardiectomy   Surgical removal of serous layer of pericardium which covers the coronary vessels and heart muscle.

Epinephrine   A hormone secreted by the adrenal medulla in response to splanchnic stimulation. The hormone is stored as granules in the gland and released in response to low blood sugar, anger, and other emotions. It is the most powerful vasopressor known—it increases blood pressure, stimulates the heart muscle, accelerates the heart rate, and increases cardiac output.

Esters   Any compound formed from an alcohol and acid by removal of water.

Excitement   The act of stimulating, arousing feelings, and provoking.

Exercise in cold weather
Patients with coronary artery disease causing myocardial ischemia do poorly in cold weather. The cold brings on angina more easily. Running for a bus in cold weather can cause a heart attack.

Fat and oils   Essential nutrients in human diets. Provides most concentrated source of energy of any foodstuff. They carry fat soluble vitamins. Principal sources of fat are meat, dairy products, poultry and fish. Principal sources of oil are nuts, vegetables and seeds. (See Cholesterol and Lipids.)

Fatty acids   Chemically edible fats consist of combinations of four molecules. Three of these are called fatty acids molecules and the fourth is glycerol (alcohol). There are tri-fatty esters of glycerol commonly called triglycerides. (*See* Esters and Triglycerides.) They differ from one another because of the various types of fatty acids they contain. All are composed of carbon, hydrogen, and oxygen atoms linked together with the carbon atoms forming the main framework of the molecule. The difference depends upon the number of carbon atoms linked together and the number of double bond carbon linkages.

Fatty acids—Monounsaturated

Are those with one double bond carbon linkage such as oleic present in most fats and oils.

Fatty acids—Polyunsaturated

Contain 2, 3 and 4 double bond carbon linkages. Because of the double bond carbon linkages these are more chemically active than saturated fatty acids. An example is *linoleic* needed in the diet with two double bond carbon linkages. It is present in most seeds, fats and vegetable oils. *Linolenic* with three double bond carbon linkages is found in soybean oil and vegetable oils. There are some polyunsaturated fatty acids with 4 or more double bonds.

Fish oils contain large quantities of a variety of longer fatty acids having three or more double bond carbon linkages.

There are both saturated and unsaturated fatty acids in most fat and oils. Those containing a high percentage of saturated fatty acids are referred to as saturated fats usually solid or semi-solid. Those with a high percentage of unsaturated fatty acids are referred to as unsaturated, and usually are liquid such as the oils.

Fatty acids—Saturated   Are

those containing only single bond carbon linkages. They are termed saturated because there are no free carbon linkages left to com-

bine with other chemicals and are the least active chemically. Examples of such are palmitic acid with 15 carbon atoms forming the chain or stearic acid with 17 carbon atoms. In both, the bond carbon linkages are single.

Fatty acids—Unsaturated   These

contain one or more double bond carbon linkages. Such fatty acids are termed unsaturated.

PERCENTAGE OF TOTAL FATTY ACIDS

Fat or Oil	Polyun- saturated fatty acids	Monoun- saturated fatty acids	Satur- ated fatty acids
Safflower Oil	75%	14%	10%
Sunflower Oil	60%	27%	11%
Soybean Oil	60%	25%	14%
Corn Oil	57%	28%	14%
Cotton Seed	46%	25%	28%
Peanut Butter	28%	50%	20%
Olive Oil	27%	50%	20%
Peanut Oil	14%	71%	14%
Lard	7%	46%	38%
Butter	tr.	33%	50%
Coconut Oil	tr.	7%	92%

Note: Margarines vary according to contents from 17% to as high as 59% polyunsaturated fatty acids in some soft vegetable oil margarines. Also, some long-chain fatty acids are not included in this chart.

Monounsaturated fatty acids have little or no effect on blood cholesterol. It is believed that polyunsaturated fatty acids do not raise the blood cholesterol, as do saturated fatty acids, but may even lower it. Thus, it is desirable to eat fats and oils with a high percentage of unsaturated fatty acids and avoid saturated fatty acids.

When substituting margarine for butter make sure that the margarine has a high percentage of unsaturated fatty acids. While good margarines contain a high percentage of unsaturated fatty acids, some contain up to 65 percent saturated fatty acids.

Fluid retention   Occurs with failure of right, left, or both ventricles.

Free omental graft   Obtained when the greater omentum is cut away from its own blood supply. When moved to another part of the body, it secretes a white substance on both its surfaces. This makes it stick to any tissue with which it comes into contact, and appears to stimulate the blood vessels of these tissues to send new branches into it. This may occur within eight days on both of its surfaces. The new blood vessels join with its vast arterial network to supply oxygenated blood to any organ, such as an ischemic heart. Through it, arterial blood may flow from the blood vessels of the pericardium to the coronary arteries.

Frequency of anginal attacks
Varies from one every few weeks to 40 daily.

Gallbladder   A pear-shaped reservoir for the bile on the undersurface of the liver. When diseased, it may cause pain in the chest similar to that of angina pectoris. It usually occurs after eating.

Greater omentum   Primitive tissue which lies between stomach and transverse colon (large bowel) from which it hangs down as a large apron covering other abdominal contents. It is rich in blood vessels, contains all types of white cells. It moves to areas of infarction (acute appendix), attempting to wall them off to prevent peritonitis. Its white cells invade, kill bacteria, and carry them away.

Heart   A muscular, four-chamber pump in the chest, lying between the lungs. It pumps unoxygenated blood from the brain, organs, glands, and muscles to the lungs for purification. From the lungs, the cleansed oxygenated (arterial) blood is pumped to every part of the body through the arteries.

Heart attack or myocardial infarction   An area of death in the heart muscle. It is due to local lack of oxygenated blood, resulting from an obstruction of coronary arterial circulation to the area.

When an area of ventricular myocardial muscle is deprived of its oxygenated blood supply, the patient usually feels chest pain (angina pectoris). This gradually disappears in a few minutes. If it persists a half hour or longer, accompanied by a cold sweat and weakness, the patient must be considered to have had a myocardial infarction, or heart attack. This occurs because the coronary artery which has been supplying an area of ventricular muscle with oxygenated blood becomes blocked, or is so narrowed that the oxygenated blood necessary to keep that portion of the ventricular muscle alive is cut off. The muscle thus dies and becomes infarcted. The patient has a myocardial infarction or heart attack.

Heart beat   Spontaneous heart muscle contraction. The heart beat first starts in the embryo and continues until death.

Heart block   Interruption of the special tissues in the Bundle of His which normally conveys impulses from the atrium which stimulate the ventricles to beat. The most common cause of interruption of the His bundle or its branches is an obstructive disease of the coronary arteries supplying the bundle. This results in reduction of cardiac rate. The cardiac rate, with sinoauricular node as pacemaker, may vary from 45 to 170 beats per minute. When the pacemaker center is shifted to the atrioventricular node, the rate may vary from 30–60 beats per minute, but it is usually 35–50 beats per minute. When the pacemaker center is shifted to one of the bundle branches, the rate is usually 20–30 beats per minute. The slowing of the heart from heart block may cause dizziness, fainting attacks, and even epileptic seizures.

Heart failure due to coronary artery insufficiency   This develops when, due to lack of adequate oxygenated blood, the heart muscle is unable to pump forward all the blood it receives. It occurs primarily in the left ventricular pump, but also in the right ventricular pump.

Heart metabolism   The heart muscle utilizes glucose, fats, amino acids, lactic acid, thiamin, nicotinic acid, riboflavin, and derivatives of Vitamin B. compound.

Heart muscle   Each heart chamber has muscle which make up its walls.

Heart muscle contraction   Heart muscle shortens when it contracts, making the heart chamber smaller and forcing blood out of the chamber.
See also Heart beat.

Heart rate   Frequency of contractions of heart muscles.

Hemoglobin   The oxygen-carrying red pigment of the red cell corpuscles. It is a reddish substance consisting of a globin protein combined with heme, an insoluble iron chemical (protoporphyrin).

Heredity   The acquisition of characters or qualities by transmission from parent to offspring.

Hiatus hernia   A defect in the left diaphragm permitting part of the stomach to slide into the chest. Pain is usually felt under the left breast.

Hypertension   Usually refers to abnormally high blood pressure.

Hysterectomy (Total)   When the ovaries as well as the uterus are removed, a premature menopause occurs. This may result in coronary atherosclerosis.

Interventricular septum   The wall separating the right and left ventricular pumps. It receives its blood supply from branches of the right and left coronary arteries. The nervous tissues in its wall conduct electrical currents to the ventricles, causing them to contract. Interference with the interventricular septum's circulation may result in heart block, requiring the introduction of an artificial pacemaker.

Isometric contraction   Contractions of skeletal muscles, which change muscle tension without muscle shortening and without approximating of its extremities.

Kinetic   Relates to motion of material bodies.

Left coronary artery   Large artery originating from the left side of the aorta. It divides into anterior descending, and circumflex coronary arteries.

Left ventricle or left ventricular pump   It is one of the four heart pumps. It receives oxygenated blood from the left atrium and pumps it out through the aorta and the entire arterial pipeline to tissues. It lies on the left side of the heart to the left of the right ventricular pump and beneath the left atrium. It has the aortic valve at its outlet into the aorta and a mitral valve between itself and the left atrium.

Left ventricular failure   When the left ventricular muscle contracts poorly, blood coming from the left atrium is not completely moved out into the aorta. This results in a backing up of blood in the left atrium and thence in the lungs. The vast capillary system in the lungs becomes congested, interfering with the oxygenation of blood. Gradually the patient becomes short of breath, requires pillows and oxygen, coughs, and may cough up clear, frothy fluid. If this persists the right ventricular pump becomes overworked and, in turn, it fails.

Leg cramps   Normally cramps may occur in the calf of the leg after hard exercise or long standing. Abnormal cramps are those which occur in the calf of a leg after walking a few blocks. They usually are due to impaired blood supply to calf muscles, caused by atherosclerosis which narrows or blocks the arteries to the legs.

Lipids   Lipids are obtained when extracting animal or vegetable tissues with one or more fat solvents; they are components of the soluble portion of the material. This includes all fats and oils. Studies have been done on the three major blood lipids: cholesterol, triglycerides and phospholipids.

Cholesterol has repeatedly been connected with clinical atherosclerotic disease. Phospholipids are said to play a protective role.

Lipoprotein   A combination of lipid and protein having the general properties of proteins. Lipids are not soluble in water. Practically all lipids of plasma are present as lipoproteins. There are two main types—alpha and beta. The beta lipoproteins transport the majority of plasma cholesterol.

Lungs   Two large air sacs on either side of the heart lying in the chest. They are connected with the mouth through the windpipe and the bronchial tubes.

Each lung is composed of thousands of small air spaces surrounded by blood capillaries. It is in the lungs that red blood cells pick up oxygen and give up carbon dioxide.

Main stem coronary artery disease   (Single, Double, and Triple) Coronary artery disease occurs throughout the surface coronary arteries. When it occurs at the origins of the arteries, it is called main stem coronary artery disease. It may occur in one, two, or three arteries, and is referred to as single, double, or triple main stem coronary artery disease. In a certain percentage of cases, it will also occur in the short main left coronary artery; if this occurs in cases with triple coronary artery disease, it is referred to as quadruple main stem coronary artery disease.

Master's two-step exercise test
This is an exercise test given to patients when the electrocardiogram is normal at rest. It consists of going up and down two steps a certain number of times in three minutes and taking an electro-

cardiographic record during the exercise. The number of steps to be performed in three minutes is determined by weight and age of the patient. Frequently, evidence of myocardial ischemia is brought out in the electrocardiogram by this test.

Metabolism   Refers to all physiological and chemical processes by which living organized substances are produced and maintained.

Morphine   The principal and most active substance in opium. Effective in relieving pain, but it is habit forming.

Myocardial arteriolar networks
A network of arterioles lying within the myocardium of right and left ventricles. They are the terminal branches of the right, anterior descending, and circumflex coronary arteries. These networks may or may not communicate with each other by collateral channels.

Myocardial arterioles   Each surface coronary artery sends branches into heart muscle where it divides into many smaller arteries called myocardial arterioles. These are the terminal divisions of branches of the surface coronary arteries within the heart muscle; they rarely become diseased.

Myocardial infarction.   *See* Heart attack.

Myocardial ischemia   Inadequate oxygenated blood supply to contracting heart muscle (myo-cardium) due to narrowing or obstruction of a coronary artery.

Narrowing coronary artery   This occurs mostly in surface coronary arteries. The narrowing is due to deposits in the artery walls. Part of the process of atherosclerosis.

Nerve endings   All nerves origi-nate from the brain and end in small twigs in the tissues. These twigs are the nerve endings. They are equipped to carry signals from the brain to every tissue in the body and to send signals back to the brain in case of trouble.

Nipple   Conelike structure which gives outlet to milk, also called the mammilla or teat.

Nitroglycerine   A drug composed of glyceryl and trinitrate. It dilates arteries, particularly coronary arteries. It is particularly effective in relieving angina pectoris, pain initiated by myocardial ischemia due to coronary artery obstruction. A small pill of nitroglycerine placed under the tongue relieves angina pectoris pain within three minutes.

Oxygenated blood.   *See* Arterial blood.

Oxyhemoglobin   Hemoglobin carrying oxygen. After picking up oxygen while passing through lungs, it is bright red (arterial). After giving up its oxygen to the tissues it turns to a purple color (venous blood).

Pacemaker—Manufactured   The first type is battery run. When the natural system of heart pacing fails, artificial pacemakers are introduced. A battery surrounded by nonirritating plastic is buried beneath the skin of the abdomen or chest. It is flat, round, about 65 mm. in diameter and 36 mm. thick. The battery sends out electrical stimuli which travel along a wire the end of which has been sutured into the muscular wall of the left ventricle. The battery can be adjusted to deliver stimuli to the heart at intervals similar to the patient's own pacing system, thus returning the pulse rate to normal. Most batteries have to be changed within 4 to 5 years.

The second type of pacemaker is the atomic. The atomic pace-maker battery is very expensive, but may last as long as 10 years. If the patient dies, it has to be recovered like other nuclear materials and disposed of.

Pacemaker nodes in heart   One pacemaker is the sino-atrial node in the wall of the right atrium, supplied by a branch of the right coronary artery and composed of specialized delicate heart fibers arranged in a snarl of connecting strands. The fibers connect with nerves and with muscle of atrium and stimulate heart contractions from 45 to 170 per minute.

The other is the atrioventricular node, a mass of specialized tissue similar to that in the sinoauricular node in the floor of right atrium, continuous above with fibers of right atrium, below with the bundle of His. When it takes control it stimulates ventricles at rates from 30–60 per minute.

Pathologist   An expert in pathology, particularly in the study of diseases after death.

Pathology   That branch of medicine which studies the essential nature of disease, especially the structural and functional changes in body tissues which cause disease or which are caused by it.

Pathology laboratories   Place equipped for investigating diseases after death.

Pectoral   Region of breast, or front of chest.

Pericardium   The fibro-serous sac that surrounds the heart. It is composed of two layers: the outer fibrous layer containing arteries which are in communication with other chest arteries; and the inner serous layer which is reflected onto and around the heart, where it covers coronary arteries, veins, and heart muscle. On the heart it is known as the epicardium. In order to permit new blood vessels to reach the heart, the serous layer of the fibrous pericardium and that covering the heart must be removed surgically. These operations are known as sero-pericardiectomy and epicardiectomy, respectively.

Persistent anginal pain   Anginal pain usually passes in a few minutes when cause is removed. Persistent anginal pain must be regarded as a myocardial infarction, i.e., heart attack, until proven otherwise.
   See also Angina pectoris. Heart attack.

Phosphatide   A fatty acid ester of a phosphorylated polyvalent alcohol.

Plasma   Fluid part of blood in which red and white cells float. It contains all the chemicals of whole blood except hemoglobin.

Pleurisy   Inflammation of the pleura which may cause recurrent chest pain.

Protein   Furnishes the raw material for growth and repair of body tissues during infancy and youth, and for repair of tissues and maintenance of body weight in adulthood.
   Proteins make up the structure of the majority of body cells. They range from the nucleoproteins in the nucleus of cells to the albumen and globulins and lipoproteins in the human plasma.
   Raw sources of protein are found in the animal and vegetable kingdoms. Proteins are the basic building blocks of human tissue. They are giant molecules which are broken down into amino acids, which in turn break down to form glucose and fatty acids.
   Proteins are the sole source of nitrogen and sulphur, and supply special amino acids for the formation of various hormones and enzymes. They supply energy and stimulate metabolism.

Revascularization surgery
Surgery performed to bring a

new source of arterial blood to those tissues lacking it due to the narrowing or blockage of the arteries which normally supply the heart. Most commonly, revascularization refers to heart muscle deprived of needed oxygenated blood, when the coronary arteries become narrowed or blocked due to atherosclerosis.

Right coronary artery This originates on the right side of the aorta, and descends on the right side of the heart. Its branches supply oxygenated blood to the muscular walls of the right atrium, the right ventricle, and to part of the division between the right and left ventricular pumping chambers. Sometimes it supplies part of the left ventricular muscle wall. In addition, it supplies the pacemakers in the heart and the nervous conduction system.

Right ventricle—right ventricular pump Receives venous (used, unoxygenated) blood from the right atrium and pumps it to the lungs for purification.

Right ventricular failure This may be secondary to left ventricular failure which causes increased pressures in the lung (against which it has to pump), thus increasing the work of the right ventricle. Occurs primarily due to lack of an adequate oxygenated blood supply to the right ventricular muscle. In either case, right ventricular failure results in swelling of the legs, enlargement of the liver, and presence of fluid in the abdomen.

Routine examination Prior to revascularization surgery, every patient should undergo a thorough examination to rule out other diseases which might influence the decision to perform surgery. A search should be made for infection in nasal sinuses, throat, teeth, gums, and in male and female urinary and genital tracts. Infections must be treated first as they are a factor in causing wound infection after surgery. Various X rays should be taken to check for a gallbladder disease which may cause trouble after surgery, peptic ulcers which may bleed, and for indications of cancer anywhere. The lungs of patients over 60 years of age should be checked most carefully for cysts, chronic bronchitis, and emphysema. Bad lungs may result in postoperative pneumonia which could throw a marginal heart into failure. The presence of severe diabetes in itself is a contra-indication to surgery, as is advanced hypertension.

Salts *Sodium:* an alkaline metallic element which in combination with chlorine is table salt.
Potassium: a metallic alkaline metal present in combination with chlorine found in orange juice and other food.
Calcium: a metallic basic element of lime. Combined with caseinate in a phosphoprotein, it is present in cows' milk.

Scar Damaged tissues heal by forming scars, much as surface wounds heal. Damaged heart muscle is replaced by scar.

Shortness of breath There are two types. First, panting with rapid breathing. Occurs normally with hard exercise and abnormally with poor lungs or failing left heart. The second type is a sensation of being unable to take a breath due to tightness of chest. This may indicate angina pectoris.

Silent heart attack (Myocardial Infarction) Many people have painless heart attacks unaccompanied by other symptoms. Thus, they are unaware of having had an attack.

Size of heart Varies with sex, body weight, height, and state of nutrition. In an average adult, it is 5 inches long, $3\frac{1}{2}$ inches wide and weighs 0.5 percent of the body weight (about 11 ounces in the male, 9 ounces in the female).

Skeletal muscles Muscles which are attached to bones, cross at least one joint, and are under voluntary control. They are responsible for body movement. Movement occurs by muscle contraction which shortens the muscle and thus the distance between two body points. In contrast, isometric contractions change the tension in muscle without approximating its extremities.

Sleeping elevated with pillows May be necessary when there is left heart failure.

Sternum The breast bone (breast plate). It lies in the front of the chest beneath the skin.

It joins above with the clavicles (collar bones) and its sides with the cartilages of the first seven ribs. It has three portions, the upper, the middle and lower which joins with the abdominal muscles.

Steroid A group name for compounds that chemically resemble cholesterol, for example, sex hormones, sterols, etc.

Sterols A solid oil. A monohydroxy alcohol of high molecular weight. One of a class of compounds widely distributed in nature which, because their solubilities are similar to those of fats, have been classified with the lipids. Cholesterol is the best known member of the group.

Stress Stress is an applied force. Strain is a response to that force.

A piece of steel is a ductile material which will deform elastically when a load is applied to it —up to a certain limit known as a *yield point* or an elastic limit. If a load less than a yield point, or stress less than a yield point, is removed, then the material returns to original size and shape.

A stress beyond the yield point causes material to deform permanently. Beyond the further limit, the material breaks. Wood does not perform like metal—the load is applied up to a certain point. Then the wood breaks without stretching.

People under stress may break like wood or yield like steel and snap back when the stress load is removed. Continued stress beyond the yield point may damage people as it does a piece of wood or steel. People under stress should remove the cause of stress if possible, learn to live with it, or remove themselves from it.

Stroke volume   The output of the left ventricle during one contraction. The stroke volume times the number of beats per minute equals cardiac output.

Sugars   Sweet carbohydrate of various kinds of both animal and vegetable origin, for example, lactose, sucrose, glucose, etc.

Surface coronary arteries   Large coronary arteries usually lie on the surface of the heart as do their surface branches. Atherosclerosis, narrowing or blocking of arteries, primarily involves the surface coronary arteries.

Surgery for coronary artery disease   (Myocardial revascularization) Coronary artery atherosclerosis narrows and blocks the coronary arteries which are the pipelines carrying the life-giving oxygenated blood to the constantly beating heart.

All operations designed to reestablish the supply of oxygenated blood to the heart muscle are called revascularization operations. There are two main types:
1. *Direct repair of coronary arteries (Pipelines to the heart)*
a. Endarterectomy—an operative procedure which scrapes out the material blocking the artery.
b. Aorto-coronary vein bypass graft—a piece of vein taken from

the thigh is sewn to a hole made in the large aorta and to a hole made in the coronary artery beyond where it is blocked.
c. Connecting the end of an internal mammary artery—after it has been freed from the chest—to a hole made in a coronary artery beyond the point of its obstruction. This operation is not to be confused with internal mammary artery implant as recommended by the author.
2. *Revascularization by indirect bypass operations—(Vineberg Operations)*
In these operations, diseased coronary arteries are not touched. Instead new arterial lines are set up to bypass the diseased coronary arteries.

a. *Implantation of the left internal mammary artery into the left ventricular wall—(Original Vineberg Operation)* In this operation, the left internal mammary artery is freed from its position beneath the chest bone and disconnected where it enters into the muscle of the abdomen. The mammary artery originates as a branch of the main artery to the arm (subclavian), and ends in the muscle of the abdomen. The end which has been separated from the abdominal muscle is pulled into a tunnel made in the wall of the left ventricle with one or two side branches bleeding, and the end tied off. It is fixed to the heart. Arterial blood escapes from the artery through its open side branches into the tunnel of the left ventricular myocardium. The blood is carried away by the myocardial sinusoidal spaces. The artery buds, which appear 12 days after surgery, and the new branches join with undiseased branches lying in the heart muscle. It is through these branches that the artery supplies the heart muscle which was deprived of its blood because of diseased surface coronary arteries.

b. *Right internal mammary artery implants into the right ventricular wall.* Procedure similar to left internal mammary artery implant, but slightly modified due to the thinness of the right ventricular wall. After implantation, the artery supplies blood to the right coronary system, and to part of the left.

c. *Implantation of right and left internal mammary arteries into right and left ventricular walls (in a single operation).* Same techniques are followed as for right and left ventricular internal mammary artery implants.

d. *Fostering the development of new vessels to supply the heart by using a free omental graft.* The greater omentum is removed from its large bowel attachment. The serous layer of the pericardium and epicardium are removed. The omentum is wrapped around the heart as a sheet, fixed in position both to the heart and to the pericardial sac.

e. *Pericoronary omental strip grafts.* Instead of using large sheets of greater omentum, the omental grafts are cut into strips containing two to three blood vessels, and each is sewn onto large surface coronary arteries. This stimulates coronary arteries to send branches into the grafts; these join with the vessels in the omentum to bypass multiple points of narrowing or occlusion caused by coronary atherosclerosis. This operation has been used in conjunction with implants. It is very recent.

Sweat   The perspiration of clear liquid from the sweat glands. Hot, normal, sweat usually occurs with normal exercise and menopause. Cold sweat comes with fear, shock, and pain.

Symptoms   Something a patient feels which may be evidence of disease.

Systolic blood pressure   Maximum arterial pressure after left ventricular contraction, averages 120 millimeters of mercury. Extremes of normal are 95 to 150 millimeters of mercury.

Tension   The condition of being stretched or strained. Working under stress causes tension and may make a person tense or tightly drawn-up. This may cause constriction of body arteries, including coronary arteries.

Thermography   A method for recording variations in temperatures (heat).

Tightness in chest   Sensation of having a steel band around the chest. Patient feels unable to take a breath. This sensation is characteristic of angina pectoris.

Treadmill A moving platform set at an angle with side rails. Used to exercise patients who walk or run in place while the platform moves continuously in a forward direction. Electrocardiograms and many other tests can be performed with the patient walking or running at different speeds. The response of his cardiovascular system to this type of exercise is evaluated.

Triglycerides (A Lipid) Ester of three fatty acids and glycerol present in fats and oils. The fatty acids may be saturated, mono-unsaturated or polyunsaturated. (*See* Fat and Oils.) They are measurable in human serum. Their elevation is considered by some as an important factor in atherosclerosis, by others it is not.

Unoxygenated blood (*See* Venous blood)

Vasopressor A hormone such as epinephrine. It stimulates contraction of muscular tissues of capillaries and arteries and raises systemic blood pressure.

Veins (*See* Blood vessels)

Venous blood Purple in color. Its red cells have given up their oxygen to the tissues.

Ventricles Large pumping chambers of heart. There are two —one on the right and the other on the left side of the heart.

Ventricular aneurysm A sac, formed by the dilatation of a wall of the ventricle (usually the left), may occur in the right ventricular wall. Most common cause is loss of blood supply to the part of the muscles making up the wall of the ventricle. This results in the death of the myocardium which is replaced by scar. In some cases the scar stretches to form a sac similar to the bulge seen in an automobile tire with a weakened wall.

Voluntary movement The muscles in the body are divided into the voluntary and the involuntary. The voluntary muscles are directly under control of the brain and spinal cord. These are the skeletal muscles that promote movement. The involuntary muscles are those that contract continuously or intermittently, such as the heart and the gastrointestinal tract. Movement in the involuntary muscles may be effected by brain stimuli, but does not depend upon the brain stimuli for action; brain stimuli are needed for voluntary movement.

Walking An exercise in which 100 percent of the body blood is moved by the heart at an increased rate. This is particularly so in the lower limbs, which contain 50 percent of the total blood volume.

Work—after heart attack
Patients with anginal pain usually continue to work unless the pain occurs very frequently. Patients after heart attack (myocardial infarction) must stop until dead heart muscle is replaced by scar in the healing process. This may take three months.

BIBLIOGRAPHY AND SOURCES

Anderson, K. Lange. *The Cardio-vascular System in Exercise.* Exercise Physiology, Harold B. Falls, Academic Press, New York and London, 1968.

Baird, R. J. *The reasons for patency and anastomosis formation of the internal mammary artery implant.* Annals of Royal College of Physicians and Surgeons of Canada, July 1969.

Baroldi, G., Scomazzoni, G. *Coronary circulation in the normal and pathological heart.* Washington Armed Forces Institute of Pathology, XV, 1967.

Beck, C. S. *The development of new blood supply to the heart by operation.* Annals of Surgery, Vol. 102, 1935.

Bigelow, W. G. *Surgical treatment of coronary heart disease.* Canadian Medical Association Journal, Vol. 104, March 20, 1971.

Campbell, J. M. H., Mitchell, G. O., and Powell, A. T. W. *Influence of Exercise on Digestion.* Guy's Hosp. Rept., Vol. 78, 1928.

Collier, W. *Functional albuminuria in athletes.* British Medical Journal, Vol. 1, 1907.

Courand, A., Ranges, H. A. *Catheterization of right auricle in man.* Proceedings Society for Experimental Biology and Medicine, Vol. 46, 1941.

Dawson, J. T., Hall, R. J., Hallman, G. L., Cooley, D. A. *Mortality in patients undergoing coronary artery bypass surgery after myocardial infarction.* American Journal of Cardiology, Vol. 33, April 1974.

Effler, Donald B. *Myocardial revascularization—direct or indirect?* Journal of Thoracic and Cardiovascular Surgery, Vol. 61, Editorial, 1971.

Effler, D. B., Favaloro, R. G., Groves, L. K., Fergusson, D. J. G. *Revascularization of left ventricle by double internal mammary artery implants.* Geriatrics, Vol. 24, April 1969.

Enos, Maj. W. F., Holmes, Col. R. H. (M.C.), Beyer, Capt. J. (M.C.). *Coronary artery disease among U.S. soldiers, killed in action in Korea.* Journal of the American Medical Association, Vol. 132, 1953.

Favaloro, R. G. *Saphenous vein autograft replacement in severe segmental artery occlusion.* Ann. Thoracic Surgery, Vol. 5, 1969.

Favaloro, R. G., Effler, D. B., Groves, L. K., Fergusson, D. J. G., Lozada, J. S. *Double internal mammary artery myocardial implantation.* Clinical Evaluation of Results in 150 Patients. Circulation, Vol. 37, April, 1968.

Forssmann, J. *Einige Immunitats-fragen im Lichte der heterogene-tischen Forschung.* Wien. klin. Wchnschr., Vol. 42, May 16, 1929.

Glenn, F., Holswade, R., Gore, A. A. *The fate of an artery implanted in the myocardium.* Surgical Forum. Clinical Congress of the American College of Surgeons, 1950.

Gordon, T., Kannel, W. B. *The effects of overweight on cardio-vascular diseases.* Geriatrics, Vol. 28, August 1973.

Green, G. E. *Direct revasculariza-tion. Internal mammary artery to left coronary artery anastomosis.* New York Journal of Medicine, Vol. 70, August 1970.

Gupta, Dwarka N. *Exercise and experimental coronary artery stricture.* Not yet in print.

Hellerstein, H. K., Friedman, E. H. *Cleveland Sexual activity and the postcoronary patient.* Archives of Internal Medicine, Vol. 125, 1970.

Humphries, J. O'Neal, Kuller, L., Ross, R. S., Friesinger, G. C., Page, E. E. *Natural history of ischemic heart disease in relation to arteriographic findings*—A twelve year study of 224 patients. Circulation, Vol. 49, March 1974.

Inter Society Commission For Heart Disease Resources. *Primary prevention of the atherosclerotic diseases.* Circulation, Vol. 42, 1970.

Johnson, W. D., Lepley, D. *An aggressive surgical approach to coronary disease.* Journal of Thoracic and Cardiovascular Surgery, Vol. 59, 1970.

Kannel, W. B., Gordon, T. *An epidemiological investigation of cardiovascular disease.* The Framingham Study. Section 28. U.S. Department of Health, Education and Welfare, Public Health Service, National Institutes of Health, DHEW Publication No. (NIH) 74-618, 1973.

Kannel, W. B., Feinleib, M., Framingham, Massachusetts, Bethesda, Maryland. *Natural history of angina pectoris in the Framingham study.* The American Journal of Cardiology, Vol. 29, February 1972.

Kannel, W. B., Schwartz, M. J., McNamara, P. M. *Blood pressure and risk of coronary heart disease.* The Framingham study. Diseases of the Chest, Vol. 56, No. 1, July 1969.

Kannel, W. B., Gordon, T. *Esti-mating risk of coronary heart disease in daily practice.* Coronary Risk Handbook, American Heart Association, New York, 1973.

Kannel, W. B., Castelli, W. P., Gordon, T., McNamara, P. M., Framingham, Massachusetts: and Bethesda, Maryland. *Serum chol-esterol, lipoproteins, and the risk of coronary heart disease.* Annals of Internal Medicine, Vol. 74, No. 1, January 1971.

Kannel, W. B. *The role of choles-terol in coronary atherogenesis.* Medical Clinics of North America, Vol. 58, No. 2, March 1974.

Kay, E. B., Suzuki, A. *Myocardial revascularization by bilateral* internal mammary artery implantation. American Journal of Cardiology, Vol. 22, 1968.

Medical Aspects of Human Sexuality, Vol. 2, No. 8, August 1972. *Heart disease and sex.* A report emanating from a series of seminars.

McKay Inc., David, New York, 1973. *American Heart Association Cookbook.*

Memorial Mercury, Vol. XII, No. 4, Winter, 1972. *Modern Medicine and Your Heart: Part I.*

O'Shaughnessy, L. *Surgical treatment of cardiac ischemia.* Lancet, Vol. 1, 1937.

Schlesinger, M. J., Zoll, P. M. *Incidence and localization of coronary occlusion.* Arch. Path., Vol. 32, 1941.

Sewell, W. H., Sones, F. M. Jr., Fish, R. G., Joyner, J. T., Effler, D. B. *The Pedicle Operation for Coronary Insufficiency: Technique and preliminary results.* Journal of Thoracic and Cardiovascular Surgery., Vol. 49, 1965.

Sones, F. M., Jr. *Heart catheterization in infancy, physiological studies.* Pediatrics, Vol. 16, October 1955.

Stinson, E. B. *Atherosclerosis in grafted heart lowered to negligible rate.* The Medical Post, January 21, 1975.

Taylor, W., Gorling, R. *Objective criteria for internal mammary artery implantation.* Ann. Thoracic Surgery, Vol. 4, 1967.

Thomas, C. B., Cohen, B. H. *The familial occurrence of hypertension and coronary artery disease, with observations concerning obesity and diabetes.* Annals of Internal Medicine, Vol. 42, 1955.

U.S. Department of Congress, 1972. *Statistical Abstract of the United States.*

Vineberg, A. M. *Development of an anastomosis between the coronary vessels and a transplanted internal mammary artery.* Canadian Medical Association Journal, Vol. 55, August, 1946.

Vineberg, A. M., Niloff, P. H. *The value of surgical treatment of coronary artery occlusion by implantation of the internal mammary artery into the ventricular myocardium.* Surgery, Gynecology and Obstetrics, Vol. 91, November 1950.

Vineberg, A. M., Miller, G. *Internal mammary coronary anastomosis in the surgical treatment of coronary artery insufficiency.* Canadian Medical Association Journal, Vol. 64, March 1951.

Vineberg, A. M., Miller, D. *Functional evaluation of an internal mammary coronary wall of the left ventricle.* Canadian Medical Association Journal, Vol. 45, April, 1953.

Vineberg, A. M. *Internal mammary artery implant in the treatment of angina pectoris. A three year follow-up.* Canadian Medical Association Journal, Vol. 70, April 1954.

Vineberg, A. M., Buller, W. *A study of the amount of blood and* oxygen delivered to the myocardium through the implanted mammary artery. Surgical Forum 5, 1955.

Vineberg, A. M., Munro, D. D., Cohen, H., Buller, W. *Four years clinical experience with internal mammary artery implantation in the treatment of human coronary insufficiency including additional experimental studies.* Journal of Thoracic Surgery, Vol. 29, January 1955.

Vineberg, A. M., Walker, J. *Six months to six years experience with coronary artery insufficiency treated by an internal mammary artery implantation.* American Heart Journal, Vol. 54, December 1957.

Vineberg, A. M., McMillan, G. C. *The fate of the internal mammary artery implant in the ischaemic human heart.* Diseases of the Chest, Vol. 33, January 1958.

Vineberg, A. M. *Internal mammary artery implantation: Survey of fifteen years of experimental study and ten years experience with human cases.* Ohio State Medical Journal, Vol. 58, October 1962.

Vineberg, A. M., Walker, J. *The surgical treatment of coronary artery heart disease by internal mammary artery implantation.* Report of 140 cases followed up to thirteen years. Diseases of the Chest, Vol. 45, February 1964.

Vineberg, A. M. *Experimental background of myocardial revas-cularization by internal mammary artery implantation and supplementary techniques, with its clinical application in 125 patients: A review and critical appraisal.* Annals of Surgery, Vol. 159, February 1964.

Vineberg, A. M., Shanks, J., Pifarre, R., Criollos, R., Kato, Y. *Combined internal mammary artery implantation and free omental graft operation: A highly effective revascularization procedure.* (A study of 17 cases). Canadian Medical Association Journal, Vol. 90, March 21, 1964.

Vineberg, A. M. *Results of 14 years experience in the surgical treatment of human coronary artery insufficiency.* Canadian Medical Association Journal, Vol. 92, February 13, 1965.

Vineberg, A. M. *Revascularization of the right and left coronary arterial systems. Internal mammary artery implantation, epicardiectomy and free omental graft operation.* The American Journal of Cardiology, Vol. 19, March 1967.

Vineberg, A. M. *Revascularization of the entire heart through myocardial arteriolar networks.* The Journal of Cardiovascular Surgery, Vol. 11, May-June 1970.

Vineberg, A. M. *Revascularization by unilateral-bilateral ventricular mammary artery implants and peri-coronary omental grafts.* Vascular Surgery, Vol. 7, No. 2, March/April 1973.

Vineberg, A. M. *The problem of blocked aorto-coronary vein grafts: Report of three cases successfully treated by intra-ventricular arterial implants and omental grafts.* The Journal of Thoracic and Cardiovascular Surgery, Vol. 66, No. 3, September, 1973.

Vineberg, A. M. *Right and left arterial implants for coronary artery insufficiency.* Paul D. White Symposium, "Major Advances in Cardiovascular Diseases," September 1973.

Vineberg, A. M., Afridi, Salim., Sahi, Sylvia. *Direct revascularization of acute myocardial infarction by implantation of left internal mammary artery into infarcted left ventricular myocardium: Preliminary experimental report.* Surgery, Gynecology & Obstetrics, Vol. 140, January 1975.

Vineberg, A. M. *Revascularization via healthy myocardial arteriolar networks compared with that through diseased surface coronary arteries.* Israel Journal of Medical Sciences Vol. II, no. 2-3, February—March 1975.

Wearn, J. T., Mettier, S. R., Klumpp, T. G., Zschiesche, L. *The nature of the vascular communications between the coronary arteries and the chambers of the heart.* Am. Heart Journal, Vol. 9, 1933.

REFERENCES DIET CHART

Feeley, Ruth M., Criner, P. E., Watt, B. K., Ph.D., R.C. Consumer and Food Economics, Research Division, Agricultural Research Service, United States Department of Agriculture, Hyattsville, Maryland. *Cholesterol Content of Foods.* Journal of the American Dietetic Association, Volume 61, August 1972.

Watt, Bernice K., Merrill, A. L., with assistance of Pecot, R. K., Adams, C. F., Orr, M. L., Miller, D. F. *Composition of Foods.* Agriculture Handbook No. 8, Consumer and Food Economics Research Division, Agricultural Research Service, United States Department of Agriculture, Washington, D.C., Revised December 1963.

Standard Brands Limited. *What's in an egg.* 1974.

Institute of Shortening and Edible Oils, Inc. *Foods Fats and Oils.* 1750 New York Avenue, N.W., Washington, D.C. 20006. August 1974